Pocket Guide to
Cardiovascular Care

Pocket Guide to
Cardiovascular Care

Susan B. Stillwell, MSN, RN, CCRN
Cleveland Clinic Foundation,
Cleveland, Ohio

Edith McCarter Randall, MS, RN, CCRN
Clinical Nurse Specialist,
St. Luke's Medical Center,
Phoenix, Arizona

Second Edition

with 77 illustrations

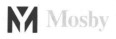

St. Louis Baltimore Boston Chicago London Madrid
Philadelphia Sydney Toronto

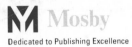

Editors: Terry Van Schaik, Timothy M. Griswold
Developmental Editor: Jolynn Gower
Project Manager: Karen Edwards
Production Editor: Gail Brower
Manufacturing Supervisor: Karen Lewis
Cover art: Jeff Holewski, Medico Graphics, Inc.

The information presented in Chapter 4 is intended as a quick reference. Information in this chapter is not intended to replace a pharmacology textbook. Detailed information and explanations are beyond the scope of this pocket guide. New information about drug therapy, contraindications, dosages, and adverse effects is ongoing. Practitioners are encouraged to read package inserts accompanying all drugs for specific manufacturer's recommendations.

Second Edition

Printed in the United States of America
Composition by Clarinda Company
Printing/binding by R.R. Donnelley & Sons Company

Mosby–Year Book, Inc.
11830 Westline Industrial Drive
St. Louis, Missouri 63146

Library of Congress Cataloging-in-Publication Data

Stillwell, Susan B.
    Pocket guide to cardiovascular care / Susan B. Stillwell, Edith
McCarter Randall.—2nd ed.
        p.   cm.
    Includes bibliographical references and index.
    ISBN 0-8016-7725-4
    1. Cardiovascular system—Diseases—Nursing—Handbooks, manuals,
etc.   I. Randall, Edith McCarter. II. Title.
    [DNLM: 1. Cardiovascular Diseases—handbooks.   WG 39 S857p   1994]
RC674.S85   1994
616. 1—dc20
DNLM/DLC
for Library of Congress   93-35578
                                                                        CIP

94 95 96 97 98   9 8 7 6 5 4 3 2 1

To my parents and my husband
for their support and belief in me.

EMR

To Paul *and* Julie
who patiently put up with me during this project;
to all students and practitioners
dedicated to provide cardiovascular care
to patients and families;
in memory of my father,
John J. Skalon.

SBS

Preface

Because cardiovascular disease is a major health care problem, health care professionals are challenged with the care of individuals regardless of their practice setting. DRGs, advances in technology and pharmacology, and the increasing necessity for home health care caused by the trend to early hospital discharges require the health care professional to evaluate the patient's health status accurately, prepare the patient for the diagnostic workup, understand sophisticated equipment, and prepare the patient to live with the disease and understand the therapeutic regimen.

The *Pocket Guide to Cardiovascular Care* is a concise, comprehensive reference. This second edition includes an update on cardiovascular problems, pharmacologic agents, and cardiovascular therapies. Information about Phase I cardiac rehabilitation and peripheral vascular surgery has been expanded. The Pocket Guide is not intended to be a textbook or a procedure manual, but rather a handy bedside reference that provides easily accessible and clinically useful information for the health care professional working in a variety of settings. Clinical Alerts, found throughout the book, highlight key points. All of these features and more make this reference an invaluable resource.

Organization of the Pocket Guide is as follows: Chapter 1, "Common Cardiovascular Problems," discusses both cardiac and vascular problems. Chapter 2, "Cardiovascular Assessment," includes major subjective and objective data, diagnostic tests, and goals of treatment. Chapter 3, "Procedures and Specialized Equipment," contains clinical guidelines related to hemodynamic monitoring, along with the description, measurement, and values for various pressures used to evaluate cardiovascular function. Also included is information about pacemakers, the IABP, the implantable cardioverter defibrillator, and cardioversion/defibrillation. Chapter 4, "Cardiovascular Pharmacologic Agents," describes drugs by classification. Administration precautions, patient assessments, and reportable adverse effects are presented. Chapter 5, "Selected Cardiovascular Therapies," examines traditional interventions such as ardiac and vascular surgery and percutaneous transluminal coronary angioplasty, and presents a review of such trends as the intravascular stent and laser therapy. Chapter 6, "Health Promotion and Home Care," reviews teaching-learning principles and includes several tables and guides for patient education and self care. The cardiac rehabilitation section provides information that is useful in facilitating self care and the transition from inpatient to outpatient. Appendices provide quick access to ACLS algorithms, administration of drugs in a cardiovascular emergency, nursing diagnoses, normal adult hemodynamic values, drug calculations, and a guide to cardiac output assessment.

We would like to express our thanks and appreciation to the editorial staff at Mosby and to the reviewers for their helpful suggestions for this second edition.

Susan B. Stillwell
Edith McCarter Randall

Contents

The rhythm strips in Chapter 2 are reprinted with permission from Conover, M.: Pocket Guide to Electrocardiography, ed. 3, St Louis, 1994, Mosby.

Common Cardiovascular Problems

1

The cardiovascular system, comprised of the heart and blood vessels, is responsible for tissue perfusion. Adequate myocardial functioning depends on normal anatomy and a balance between myocardial oxygen supply and demand (Table 1-1). Myocardial oxygen supply is greatest during diastole but the demand on the heart is greatest during systole. Figure 1-1 depicts both the mechanical and electrical events of one cardiac cycle.

An intact vascular system transports blood to and from tissues. Despite an adequate cardiac output, tissue perfusion may be impaired if a condition exists that affects the patency of blood vessels.

Alterations in heart and blood vessel structures and an imbalance in myocardial oxygen supply and demand are major causes of cardiovascular dysfunction. This chapter presents an overview of select cardiovascular problems and treatments.

Coronary Artery Disease

Overview

Coronary artery disease (CAD) is a disease process characterized by atherosclerotic plaque, a buildup of lipids primarily within the intimal layer of the coronary arteries. The atherosclerotic lesions begin in childhood as fatty streaks and progress to fibrous plaque and, finally, to the advanced or complicated lesion. These lesions cause narrowing of the arterial lumen and consequently reduce or obstruct myocardial blood flow.

Multiple risk factors have been linked to atherosclerosis. Non-modifiable risk factors include age, sex, race, and heredity. Major

Table 1-1   Determinants of myocardial oxygen supply and demand

Oxygen Supply	
Coronary blood flow	
Oxygen extraction by myocardial cells	
Oxygen Demand	
Preload	Volume in ventricle at end diastole; reflected by CVP, PAD, PAW, LA pressures
Afterload	Resistance the ventricle pumps against; reflected by SVR, PVR
Contractility	Ability of muscle fibers to shorten; reflected by LVSWI, RVSWI
Heart rate	Number of ventricular contractions per minute; reflected by pulse rate, ECG

CVP, central venous pressure. PAD, pulmonary artery diastolic. PAW, pulmonary artery wedge. LA, left atrial. SVR, systemic vascular resistance. PVR, pulmonary vascular resistance. LVSWI, left ventricular stroke work index. RVSWI, right ventricular stroke work index. ECG, electrocardiogram.

modifiable risk factors that can be altered through changes in lifestyle and the use of pharmacologic agents include cigarette smoking, high blood pressure, and elevated cholesterol levels. Contributory factors include physical inactivity, obesity, glucose intolerance, stress, and hormones.

Cigarette smoking causes an increase in heart rate and myocardial oxygen consumption secondary to increased catecholamine release, a reduction in the oxygen-carrying capacity of the blood secondary to the production of carbon monoxide, and changes in lipoproteins that contribute to CAD. Increased platelet adhesiveness and potential thrombus formation have also been implicated with cigarette smoking.

High blood pressure causes injury or structural damage to vessels and also results in left ventricular hypertrophy. There is an increased prevalence of high blood pressure in individuals with glucose intolerance and in those who are overweight.

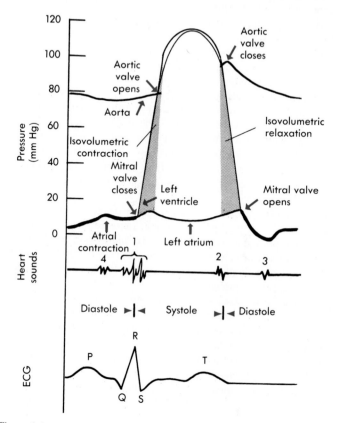

Figure 1-1
Events of the cardiac cycle. Electrical depolarization of the ventricle (represented by the QRS) precedes mechanical systole (contraction), which begins with the first heart sound (S_1) and ends with the second heart sound (S_2). The amount of blood ejected with one contraction (stroke volume) times the number of contractions per minute (heart rate) determines the cardiac output for one minute.

Elevated levels of low-density lipoprotein (LDL) associated with obesity and smoking promotes atherosclerosis, whereas increased levels of high-density lipoprotein (HDL) serve as protectors from the atherosclerotic process. A decrease in HDL increases the risk of CAD and is associated with individuals who smoke, are physically inactive, and are overweight.

CAD may cause angina, myocardial infarction (MI), and heart failure. Since individuals with heart disease can range from being asymptomatic to being totally disabled, a thorough cardiac appraisal should be done. Criteria for evaluating heart disease have been established by the New York Heart Association (Table 1-2) and are widely used to determine a patient's cardiac status and prognosis. Etiologic, anatomic, and physiologic diagnoses are used to evaluate the patient's cardiac status, and prognosis is based on the potential effects of the various medical and surgical therapies available.

Angina is a subjective experience that the patient may express as "pressure," "crushing," or "burning" retrosternal discomfort or a sensation of "tightness," "achiness," or "indigestion" in the chest. Chest discomfort may not always be localized but may radiate to the jaw or arms. Still, some patients are asymptomatic during myocardial ischemic episodes.

Myocardial ischemia is caused by an imbalance in the myocardial oxygen supply and demand (see Table 1-1). In some patients, a fixed (atherosclerotic) lesion that obstructs 50% of the coronary arterial lumen can produce angina when the demand on the heart is increased (i.e., with activity). In other patients, a 75% to 100% obstruction may be present before angina is experienced. Vasospasm may be the cause of angina when demands on the heart are con-

Table 1-2   New York Heart Association classification of heart disease

Cardiac Status	Prognosis
I. Uncompromised	Good
II. Slightly compromised	Good with therapy
III. Moderately compromised	Fair with therapy
IV. Severely compromised	Guarded despite therapy

From the Criteria Committee of the New York Heart Association, Nomenclature and criteria for diagnosis of diseases of the heart and great vessels, ed 8, 1979.

stant (i.e., at rest). Coronary vasospasm can occur both in patients with normal coronary arteries and in patients with fixed lesions. Descriptions of various types of angina can be found in Table 1-3, and a commonly used grading system for effort angina is described in Table 1-4.

Prolonged ischemia results in acute myocardial infarction. The lack of oxygen supply to the myocardium, which usually results from a thrombus formation in a coronary artery, causes ischemia, injury, and death to the area of the myocardium supplied by the occluded artery. Other precipitating factors include coronary vasospasm and platelet aggregation. Cocaine, a cardiac stimulant, has

Table 1-3   **Classifications of angina**

Type	Description
Stable (classic, effort, or exertional angina)	Precipitating factor can be identified. Relieved within 2-5 minutes with rest or nitroglycerin. Fixed lesion impedes blood flow, attacks are similar, relief is obtained by the same intervention.
Unstable (preinfarction, crescendo, coronary insufficiency)	Stable angina that has changed in quality, frequency, intensity, duration, or timing. Pain is difficult to control. Patients are at risk for myocardial infarction or sudden death.
Variant (Prinzmetal's, coronary vasospasm)	Occurs at rest. ST elevation on ECG during chest discomfort is a hallmark.
Mixed Angina	Combination of exertional angina and coronary vasospasm.
Nocturnal	Occurs during sleep and awakens the patient.
Decubitus	Occurs while patient is resting in a supine position.

Table 1-4   Canadian Cardiovascular Society grading system for effort angina

Grade	Activity Limitation	Angina Occurs With
1	None	Exertion at work or play that is strenuous, rapid, or prolonged.
2	Slight	Walking: rapidly, uphill, after meals, in cold weather, in the wind, under emotional stress, after a few hours of awakening, more than 2 blocks. Climbing stairs: rapidly, after meals, in cold weather, in the wind, under emotional stress, more than 1 flight of ordinary stairs at a normal pace, under normal conditions.
3	Marked	Walking: 1-2 level blocks. Climbing: 1 flight of stairs at a normal pace, under normal conditions.
4	Severe	Any physical activity; may be present at rest.

Modified from Campeau L: Grading of angina pectoris (letter), *Circulation* 54:522, 1976.

also been implicated as a causative agent in myocardial infarctions. An infarction consists of three areas or zones that are associated with alterations in function and electrophysiology. The center zone consists of necrotic tissue and is electrically inert. Pathologic Q waves on ECG are reflective of this zone. Immediately adjacent to this zone is the area of injury, which is undergoing metabolic changes and is electrophysiologically unstable. ST segments in the leads over the injured area are elevated on ECG. An ischemic area, which is also undergoing metabolic alterations and is electrically unstable, surrounds the injury zone. Both the necrotic and injury areas are noncontractile and therefore affect left ventricular function. Impaired left ventricular function results in a decreased stroke volume, stroke work, cardiac output, and ejection fraction and increases end diastolic ventricular pressures. The electrical instability present in the injured and ischemic areas predispose the patient to dysrhythmias, the most common complication following MI.

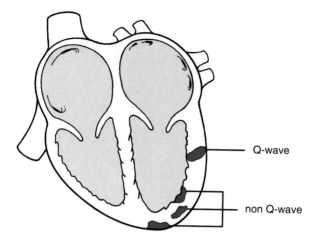

Figure 1-2
Types of infarctions.

There are two major types of infarctions: Q wave infarction (transmural), in which the full thickness of the ventricular wall is affected, and non–Q wave infarctions (nontransmural) (Figure 1-2). Non–Q wave infarctions can be further subdivided into subendocardial, subepicardial, and intramural infarctions. The location of infarctions depends on which coronary artery is occluded (Table 1-5; also see Table 2-20).

Within 24 hours of a myocardial infarction, cardiac enzymes are released into the bloodstream, and leukocytes infiltrate the infarcted area in response to the inflammatory process. Glycogenolysis and lipolysis occur with infarction, elevating serum glucose levels. The necrotic tissue is removed by the third day, and the area is replaced with scar tissue in its beginning form. After 2 weeks scar tissue is still weak, and it will replace all necrotic tissue within 4 to 6 weeks.

Major Subjective/Objective Data

The patient's major complaint, and possibly the first symptom of CAD, is chest pain or discomfort that increases in intensity and then gradually subsides (see Table 2-2). The event precipitating an-

Table 1-5 Overview of coronary arteries

	RCA	LCx	LAD
Major areas supplied	RA, RV, inferior LV, portion of ventricular septum	LA, lateral and posterior LV wall	Anterior wall of LV, apex, portion of septum
Conduction system supplied	SA node,* AV node,† His bundle‡	SA node, AV node, His bundle	Right bundle, left bundle
Major effect if occluded	RV infarction, inferior MI, disturbances of upper conduction system (sinus bradycardia, second degree AV block Mobitz type I), ventricular ectopy	Lateral MI, ventricular ectopy	Anterior MI, disturbances of lower conduction system (BBB, second-degree AV block Mobitz type II, third-degree heart block), ventricular ectopy, pump disturbance

RCA, right coronary artery. SA, sinoatrial. LCx, left circumflex. AV, atrioventricular. LAD, left anterior descending. RA, right atrium. RV, right ventricle. LA, left atrium. LV, left ventricle. BBB, bundle branch block.
*In 55% of the population.
†In 80% of the population.
‡In 90% of the population.

Table 1-6   Classification of acute myocardial infarction

Class	Failure	Manifestations
I	None	None
II	Mild-moderate	Sinus tachycardia, S_3, crackles
III	Acute pulmonary edema	Extreme dyspnea; anxiety; pallor; cyanosis; cool, clammy skin
IV	Cardiogenic shock	Systolic BP <80 mm Hg; thready pulse; cool, clammy skin; cyanosis; restlessness and confusion

From Killip T, Kimball J: Treatment of myocardial infarction in a coronary care unit, *American Journal of Cardiology* 20:459, 1967

gina may be known, and the physical examination may or may not be normal. Associated signs and symptoms may include nausea or vomiting, dyspnea, diaphoresis, increased blood pressure and pulse, and dysrhythmias.

Prolonged angina that is unrelieved by nitroglycerin may be indicative of an MI. In some cases, chest pain is absent and the "silent MI" may be recognized only on routine ECG. Clinical manifestations may vary depending on the degree of myocardial dysfunction. A classification of acute MI, based on left ventricular function, has been used to determine the patient's prognosis (Table 1-6). Prognosis worsens as the patient develops signs and symptoms characteristic of class III or IV.

Diagnostic Tests

Since coronary atherosclerosis has been associated with lipid accumulation, serum lipid levels should be evaluated. Both low-density and high-density lipoproteins are risk predictors of CAD. Lipoproteins depend on apolipoproteins for metabolism and lipid transfer, thus any disorder in lipoproteins can be related to an alteration in the structure or function of apolipoproteins. Apolipoproteins A-I (an HDL component) and B (an LDL component) are thought to be more discriminating than serum lipids in predicting coronary heart disease.

In addition to screening individuals for elevated cholesterol levels, tests are used to differentiate between ischemia and infarction

Table 1-7   Diagnostic tests commonly used in patients with coronary artery disease

Test	Comment
ECG	Helpful in variant angina: ST elevation during chest discomfort; dysrhythmias may be present. Abnormal Q waves, ST elevation, and T wave changes present in leads over the infarcted area. (See Table 2-19.)
Ambulatory monitor	ST segment depression or elevation can be documented. Silent ischemia and dysrhythmias can be documented.
Exercise ECG	ST depression within 3 minutes of exercise, persistent ST segment depression 8 minutes after exercise; downward sloping or 1 mm or greater ST depression lasting 0.08 second; and hypotension are indicators of a positive test. Less helpful in vasospasm.
Serum lipids	Elevated total cholesterol and LDL levels contribute to CAD. A low HDL level is also a risk for CAD. A total cholesterol/HDL ratio >4.5 increases the risk of CAD.
Cardiac enzymes	A characteristic pattern is diagnostic of MI; CK-MB is specific for myocardial damage; LDH flip is indicative of MI. (See Tables 2-11 and 2-12.)
Serum myoglobin	Elevated in MI patients within 1 hour after the MI.
Echocardiography	Abnormal wall movement may be present. Used to evaluate valvular function and measure ejection fraction.
Radionuclide imaging studies	Thallium scan "cold spots" suggest ischemia or old infarction.

Table 1-7   Diagnostic tests commonly used in patients with coronary artery disease—cont'd

Test	Comment
Cardiac catheterization and coronary arteriography	Technetium 99m "hot spots" indicate acute infarction.
	Positron emission tomography identifies ischemia and infarcted areas.
	Abnormal movement (i.e., dyskinesia, akinesia, hypokinesia, asyneresis, asynchrony) may be present with ischemic attacks.
	Coronary arteries are visualized and stenotic areas identified.
	Spasm may be diagnosed if ergonovine maleate test is positive.

and to evaluate the effects of CAD on myocardial functioning (Table 1-7).

Refer to Chapter 2 for additional information on diagnostic tests.

Treatment

Prevention of CAD requires education on risk factors and methods to reduce them (see Chapter 6). Medical treatment includes drug therapy aimed at reducing the oxygen demand on the heart and increasing the blood supply to the myocardium. Combination therapy is commonly used. Nitrates are used to lower myocardial workload by decreasing preload and afterload. Short-acting nitrates are used during an acute attack and can be used prophylactically before any known activity that causes angina. Caution should be used with the administration of nitrates to patients with inferior or right ventricular infarctions, since a sudden drop in blood pressure and heart rate may occur. Beta adrenergic blocking agents are used early in the acute MI to reduce myocardial workload and have been shown to reduce mortality after MI. These agents reduce heart rate and decrease contractility, thereby decreasing myocardial oxygen consumption. Calcium channel blocking agents are used to decrease afterload, heart rate, and contractility and to improve oxygen supply by dilating coronary arteries. Aspirin is prescribed to reduce platelet aggregation and prevent myocardial reinfarction. Antihyperlipidemic agents may be prescribed to reduce serum lipid levels when dietary modifications have failed.

Controversy exists over routine consumption of fish oil tablets to retard atherosclerosis. Fish oils containing omega-3 fatty acids have antiplatelet effects, lower total cholesterol levels, reduce arterial pressure, decrease whole blood viscosity, and increase erythrocyte deformability. Adverse effects include bleeding, altered immune system function, and increased cholesterol levels with low and moderate doses (approximately 8 g of fish oil is needed per day to obtain beneficial effects).

Left ventricular function may be assessed in patients with acute MI via a pulmonary artery catheter. Hemodynamic parameters, which are helpful to evaluate the patient's response to therapy, can be continuously monitored at the bedside. The pulmonary artery wedge pressure reflects compliance of the left ventricle and its ability to empty; an increase in pressure is associated with left ventricular impairment.

Invasive procedures to treat CAD may include percutaneous transluminal coronary angioplasty, thrombolytic therapy, and revascularization surgery, all of which are discussed in Chapter 5.

Patients experiencing unstable angina or manifestations of acute MI are admitted to the coronary care unit, placed on continuous ECG monitoring, have a venous access established, and are given oxygen therapy. Other commonly employed interventions can be found in Table 1-8.

Complications of MI are numerous (Table 1-9), with dysrhythmias being the most common. A late complication is Dressler's syndrome (characterized by pericarditis with effusion and fever), which is thought to be a result of an antigen-antibody reaction. Heart failure can also result from right or left ventricular infarctions. Although right ventricular infarctions are rare, they should not be confused with right-sided heart failure. Administering diuretics (a common practice in heart failure) should be avoided in patients with right ventricular infarction, since a further reduction in cardiac output may result. Volume expansion is needed to improve hypotension associated with right ventricular infarction.

Cardiogenic shock is generally associated with an acute myocardial infarction where there is loss of more than 40% of ventricular muscle. The reduced cardiac output and low blood pressure

Table 1-8 **Interventions and rationale for patients with unstable angina or acute myocardial infarction**

Intervention	Rationale
IV morphine sulfate	Reduces workload on heart by decreasing chest discomfort, preload, afterload, and stress.
IV nitroglycerin	Decreases chest discomfort unrelieved by narcotics; decreases preload and afterload, which reduces myocardial oxygen demand.
Antidysrhythmics	Abolish or control dysrhythmias and thereby improve cardiac output. Lidocaine may be used prophylactically.
Antihypertensives	Decrease afterload and thus reduce myocardial oxygen demand.
Diuretics	Decrease preload and afterload and thus reduce the workload on the heart; however, they may compromise cardiac output further in patients with inferior MI (hypervolemia may not be involved—fluid status must be assessed).
Heparin	Prophylactic anticoagulation with low-dose heparin.
Beta adrenergic blockers	Prophylaxis for myocardial reinfarction; treatment of dysrhythmias; reduce heart rate and thus myocardial oxygen demand.
Calcium channel blockers	Decrease coronary vasospasm, reduce blood pressure, and control dysrhythmias.
Antiplatelet agents	Prophylaxis for myocardial reinfarction.
Tranquilizers	Decrease anxiety (decreases SNS effects and thus decreases oxygen demand).
Stool softeners	Prophylaxis for constipation (reduces the risk of the effects of the Valsalva maneuver).
Activity restriction	Reduces workload on heart.

Continued.

Table 1-8   Interventions and rationale for patients with unstable angina or acute myocardial infarction—cont'd

Intervention	Rationale
Diet restriction	Soft diet to aid digestion, salt restriction to reduce fluid retention, and cholesterol restriction to retard atherosclerotic process.
Counterpulsation	Provides temporary reduction in myocardial oxygen consumption and improvement in coronary artery perfusion.
Angioplasty	Relieves the obstruction to blood flow in a stenosed coronary artery by flattening plaque with an inflated balloon.
Thrombolytic therapy	Salvages myocardium by lysing coronary artery thrombi and restoring coronary blood flow
Revascularization	Circumvents an obstruction in a coronary artery by using a saphenous vein or internal mammary artery. Multiple grafts may be implanted depending on the extent of disease, coronary anatomy, and availability of graft material.

contribute to decreased coronary artery blood flow, which further increases myocardial ischemia and necrosis. This further impairs contractility, and thus a vicious cycle continues. The mortality rate for patients developing cardiogenic shock is 75% to 90%.

Priorities of care include pain assessment and management, evaluation of the patient's hemodynamic response to therapy, and early detection of complications. Interventions to reduce workload on the heart should be implemented (decrease stress and anxiety, initiate bedrest if symptomatic or if complications develop, use bedside commode, reduce pain).

Patient education regarding risk factors, dietary changes, activities, medications, precipitating factors, and signs and symptoms that require immediate medical attention is critical to promoting cardiovascular health. (See Chapter 6.)

Table 1-9 Complications following myocardial infarction

Problem	Treatment
Dysrhythmias (see Chapter 2)	
Sinus tachycardia	Remove cause (i.e., pain, anxiety)
Atrial flutter	Drug therapy (i.e., digoxin, quinidine, verapamil) Cardioversion Overdrive pacing
Atrial fibrillation	Drug therapy (i.e., digoxin, verapamil, propranolol, quinidine, procainamide) Cardioversion
Bradycardia	Drug therapy (i.e., atropine, isoproterenol) Pacemaker
Heart block (2nd-degree AV block type II; 3rd-degree block)	Pacemaker
Ventricular tachycardia (VT)	Drug therapy (i.e., lidocaine, procainamide, bretylium tosylate) Cardioversion
Ventricular fibrillation or pulseless VT	Defibrillate
Other Complications	
Heart failure	Drug therapy: inotropes (i.e., digoxin, dobutamine, amrinone); diuretics (i.e., furosemide, if indicated [based on volume status]); vasodilators (i.e., nitroprusside, nitroglycerin, prazosin), ACE inhibitors, (i.e., enalapril maleate, captopril) Fluid restriction
Cardiogenic shock	Drug therapy: inotropes (i.e., dobutamine, dopamine); vasodilators (i.e., nitroprusside, nitroglycerin) IABP

Continued.

Table 1-9   Complications following myocardial
infarction—cont'd

Problem	Treatment
Papillary muscle rupture	Drug therapy: vasodilators (i.e., nitroprusside) Mitral valve replacement IABP
Rupture of interventricular septum	IABP Surgical repair
Left ventricular wall rupture	Surgical repair
Ventricular aneurysm	Anticoagulation with heparin Aneurysmectomy
Pericarditis	Drug therapy (i.e., aspirin, indomethacin, corticosteroids)
Dressler's syndrome	Drug therapy (i.e., aspirin, indomethacin, corticosteroids)

IABP, intraaortic balloon pump.

Clinical Alert

During an acute ischemic attack, have the patient stop the activity, administer oxygen and nitroglycerin or a narcotic, take vital signs, obtain an ECG if ordered, and stay with the patient.

The onset of tachycardia, S_3, and crackles are common manifestations of left ventricular failure (see "Cardiac Failure" later in this chapter).

A sustained arterial blood pressure < 90 mm Hg in a previously normotensive person accompanied by evidence of inadequate tissue perfusion (cold, clammy skin; thready, weak pulses; change in sensorium) may indicate cardiogenic shock. Pharmacologic agents along with intraaortic balloon counterpulsation may be required.

Cardiac Failure

Overview

Cardiac failure is a term that is synonymous with heart failure, cardiac decompensation, congestive heart failure, and the failing heart. It is a state in which the heart is unable to adequately supply blood to meet the metabolic needs of the body. Common causes of car-

Table 1-10   Contributing factors to cardiac failure

Condition	Mechanism
Anemia Fever Hypoxemia Hyperthyroidism Stress Tachydysrhythmias	Produce tachycardia, which increases myocardial oxygen consumption and decreases diastolic filling.
Cardiac depressant drugs Cardiomyopathy Hypoxemia Acidosis	Decrease contractility, which results in a reduced cardiac output.
Polycythemia Fluid overload	Increase preload and afterload, which increases myocardial work.

diac failure include hypertension, valvular disease, congenital heart disease, coronary artery disease, myocardial infarction, and cardiomyopathies. Conditions that may precipitate cardiac failure are presented in Table 1-10.

The physiologic abnormalities in heart failure are a reduction in cardiac output and elevated ventricular end diastolic filling pressures. When cardiac output (CO) decreases, the heart attempts to compensate by increasing the heart rate. However, tachycardia impairs ventricular filling because the time between beats (diastole) is decreased.

Stroke volume depends on preload, afterload, and contractility. As end diastolic pressure (preload) increases within physiologic limits, myocardial fibers are stretched and contraction is stronger, resulting in increased stroke volume (Starling's law). However, in heart failure, an increase in preload does not result in increased stroke volume. Myocardial fibers are stretched beyond the optimal length for forceful contractions, and consequently the ventricles' contractility is impaired. If afterload is increased, as with hypertension, the failing heart's pumping ability is further compromised. Thus stroke volume and cardiac output decrease even further.

A reduced stroke volume results in an increase in the amount of blood that remains in the ventricles, raising diastolic (ventricular) filling pressures. When left ventricular filling pressure increases, the left atrial pressure also increases. This pressure is reflected in the pulmonary circulation and is the cause for the major subjective and objective findings of left-sided heart failure. Manifestations of right-sided heart failure are reflective of increased systemic venous pressures. Although right-sided heart failure can occur secondary to pulmonary disease, the primary cause of right-sided heart failure is left-sided failure (Figure 1-3).

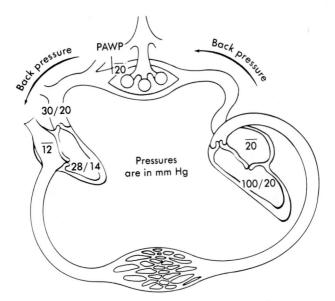

Figure 1-3
Right and left ventricular heart failure. An increase in left ventricular end-diastole and left atrial pressures leads to increased pulmonary artery wedge and pulmonary artery pressures. These pressures cause pulmonary capillary fluid leakage, causing pulmonary signs and symptoms associated with left-sided heart failure. Right ventricular failure results from the increased pulmonary artery pressures. The increased pressures of the right side of the heart cause fluid to leak from the capillaries in the systemic circulation, producing peripheral edema.
From Quaal S: *Comprehensive intra-aortic balloon counterpulsation*, St Louis, 1993, Mosby.

A reduced cardiac output can cause a decrease in organ perfusion and consequently affect the patient's sensorium, myocardial oxygen supply, and kidney function. When the kidneys are underperfused, the renin-angiotensin-aldosterone system is stimulated. This reaction causes vasoconstriction (increased afterload) and sodium and water retention (increased preload). Although this is a compensatory mechanism, the end result increases myocardial workload and further compromises ventricular function in an already failing heart.

An acute manifestation of left ventricular failure is pulmonary edema. This condition can be life-threatening and results from increased pulmonary venous pressure secondary to the decreased pumping ability of the left ventricle. The high pulmonary hydrostatic pressure exceeds plasma oncotic pressure and rapidly forces fluid into the alveoli, impairing gas exchange. Patients are acutely short of breath, restless and extremely anxious, and diaphoretic. Patients are "drowning" in their own fluid and may exhibit orthopnea, tachypnea, frothy pink sputum, and cyanosis.

Major Subjective/Objective Data

The clinical manifestations of heart failure are related to the increased pressure in the pulmonary and peripheral venous circulation and to reduced cardiac output (Table 1-11).

Diagnostic Tests

Abnormal laboratory results reflecting hepatic or renal impairment may be a result of decreased organ perfusion or increased venous pressure. BUN and creatinine are usually mildly elevated, hyponatremia may be present, and liver function values may be elevated. Other diagnostic tests can be used to determine the cause or degree of heart failure but are not required or diagnostic for heart failure. The ECG may show abnormalities such as dysrhythmias, chamber enlargement, and left ventricular hypertrophy, as a result of the underlying cardiac disease. Radionuclide studies and echocardiogram are helpful to evaluate wall motion and ejection fraction and can be helpful in the search for the cause of heart failure, for example, a valvular disorder. Cardiac catheterization is rarely performed to diagnose heart failure, but it can provide added information about ventricular filling pressures and cardiac output. Refer to Chapter 2 for additional information on cardiovascular diagnostic tests.

Table 1-11   Possible clinical manifestations of cardiac failure

Signs Associated with Right-sided Heart Failure

Nausea	Increase in RAP, CVP
Anorexia	Jugular venous distention
Weight gain	+ hepatojugular reflex
Ascites	Right ventricular heave
Right upper quadrant pain	Murmur of tricuspid insufficiency
	Hepatomegaly
	Peripheral edema

Signs Associated with Left-sided Heart Failure

Fatigue	Tachycardia
Cough	S$_3$ gallop
Shortness of breath	Crackles
DOE	Increased PAP, PAWP, SVR
Orthopnea	Laterally displaced PMI
PND	Left ventricular heave
Diaphoresis	Pulsus alternans
	Confusion
	Decreased urine output
	Cheyne-Stokes respirations (advanced failure)
	Murmur of mitral insufficiency

RAP, right atrial pressure. CVP, central venous pressure. PAP, pulmonary artery pressure. PAWP, pulmonary artery wedge pressure. SVR, systemic vascular resistance. DOE, dyspnea on exertion. PND, paroxysmal nocturnal dyspnea. PMI, point of maximal impulse.

Treatment

Elimination or prompt treatment of precipitating cause(s) is important when managing the patient with a failing heart. The administration of ACE inhibitors to patients with asymptomatic left ventricular dysfunction can reduce the incidence of overt heart failure and improve prospects for survival. Ultimately, therapy is aimed at improving cardiac output without increasing the workload on the heart. A typical treatment plan includes oxygen administration, a balanced activity and rest program, weight reduction if necessary, fluid and electrolyte management, pharmacologic agents (see box

Pharmacologic Agents that Manipulate Determinants of Cardiac Output*

Agents that Increase Contractility

Cardiac glycosides (i.e., digoxin)
Phosphodiesterase inhibitors (i.e., amrinone, milrinone)
Sympathomimetics (i.e., dobutamine, dopamine)

Agents that Reduce Preload

Diuretics (i.e., furosemide, bumetanide)
Balanced vasodilators (i.e., nitroprusside)

Agents that Reduce Afterload

Antihypertensives (i.e., hydralazine)
Angiotensin-converting enzyme inhibitors (i.e., captopril, enalapril maleate)
Balanced vasodilators (i.e., nitroprusside sodium)

Agents that Regulate Heart Rate

Antidysrhythmic agents (i.e., verapamil)
Cardiac glycosides (i.e., digoxin)

*Refer to Chapter 4 for additional information on drugs.

above), counterpulsation if necessary, and surgery if indicated (valve replacement, commissurotomy, or heart transplant). Hemodynamic monitoring with a pulmonary artery catheter is helpful to assess the patient's left ventricular function and evaluate the patient's response to therapy (see Appendix C).

A patient in cardiac failure requires careful assessment of cardiac output; early detection of complications, such as pulmonary edema and digitalis intoxication; accurate fluid and electrolyte management; and education regarding the condition and therapeutic regimen.

Clinical Alert

To prevent fluid volume overload in patients with heart failure, do not administer normal saline solutions.

Increased respiratory effort, hypoxemia, pink frothy sputum,

Table 1-12 Comparison of cardiomyopathies

Disorder	Primary Feature	Comment
Dilated (DC)	Ventricular dilatation; impaired systolic function	Most common. Both ventricles are dilated. Emboli may occur secondary to stasis of blood in the dilated ventricles.
Hypertrophic (HC)	Inappropriate myocardial hypertrophy; nondilated left ventricle	May or may not be obstructive. Obstructive type has been previously referred to as idiopathic hypertrophic subaortic stenosis (IHSS). Ventricular cavity may be normal or decreased; outflow tract obstruction is caused by the hypertrophied septum and displaced mitral valve. Ventricular compliance is decreased and thus diastolic filling is impaired.
Restrictive (RC)	Decreased diastolic compliance	Least common; ventricular cavity size is decreased; disease process results in fibrosis of myocardium. Clinical manifestations are similar to constrictive pericarditis.

and crackles are signs and symptoms of pulmonary edema. Be prepared to administer morphine and diuretics and possibly apply rotating tourniquets to decrease the circulating volume. Supplemental oxygen by mask or intubation with mechanical ventilation may be required.

Cardiomyopathies

Overview

Cardiomyopathies, disorders of the structure and function of the myocardium, are classified into three major groups: dilated (congestive), hypertrophic, and restrictive. The primary features of these disorders are identified in Table 1-12. They can be further classified into primary (idiopathic) or secondary (a result of another abnormality) cardiomyopathies. Figure 1-4 shows a comparison of the cardiomyopathies during the cardiac cycle.

Dilated cardiomyopathy (DC) is the most common. Infection, metabolic abnormalities, and toxic substances have been implicated

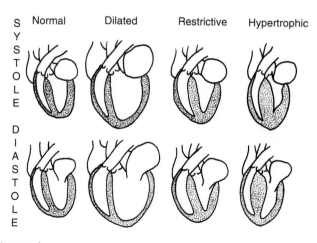

Figure 1-4
Types of cardiomyopathies.
Modified from Goldman M, Boucher C: *Am J Cardiol* 46:1235, 1980.

as causative factors in DC. Prognosis is poor because heart failure, the major complication, becomes increasingly difficult to treat. Pulmonary emboli are also common.

Hypertrophic cardiomyopathy (HC) may or may not be associated with an obstruction of the left ventricular outflow tract. Cardiac output can be adversely affected in patients with the obstructive lesion. Heredity has been implicated as a causative factor in HC. Sudden death may be the first manifestation of the disease. Development of atrial fibrillation is a poor prognostic sign. Diastolic filling is already impaired in HC and a loss of atrial kick and rapid ventricular response of atrial fibrillation can further compromise cardiac output. Ventricular dysrhythmias are common. Embolization can also occur in patients with HC.

Restrictive cardiomyopathy (RC) is rare and resembles constrictive pericarditis. Endomyocardial fibrosis has been cited as the most common cause of RC. The right and/or left ventricles may be involved, although patients predominantly exhibit the signs of right ventricular failure. Cardiac output is decreased since the myocardium is rigid and ventricular filling is impaired.

Major Subjective/Objective Data

Generally, patients will manifest signs and symptoms of heart failure, dysrhythmias, conduction disturbances, or sudden death.

Clinical manifestations of DC include the following: pale, cool skin; hypodynamic and laterally displaced apical pulse; dysrhythmias; crackles; holosystolic murmurs of tricuspid and mitral regurgitation; S_3 and S_4; summation gallop; and signs of right-sided heart failure in end stage disease. Patients may experience fatigue, dyspnea, orthopnea, and cough.

Clinical manifestations of HC include a systolic ejection murmur that often radiates to the lower sternum, both axillae, and base of heart; systolic thrill at the fourth interspace, left sternal border; and an arterial pulse that is brisk, abrupt, and poorly sustained. Patients may experience fatigue, dyspnea, chest pain or discomfort, dizziness, or syncope.

Clinical manifestations of RC include signs of right-sided and left-sided heart failure (right side usually predominates), dysrhythmias, S_3 and S_4, murmurs of tricuspid and mitral regurgitation, and pulsus paradoxus. Patients may experience fatigue, fever, dyspnea, and chest pain or discomfort.

Diagnostic Tests

Diagnosing cardiomyopathies is challenging because these disorders mimic other cardiovascular conditions. The tests reveal findings consistent with heart failure and the presence or absence of hypertrophy (Table 1-13). As with other cardiovascular disorders, these tests can also be used to evaluate the patient's response to therapy. Refer to Chapter 2 for additional information on cardiovascular diagnostic tests.

Treatment

Medical and surgical intervention may be required to control symptoms. However, prognosis for patients with a cardiomyopathy is poor.

The treatment for DC is focused on improving cardiac index without adversely reducing ventricular filling pressures (dilated ventricles require higher filling pressures to maintain an acceptable cardiac output). Positive inotropic agents (dobutamine and dopamine) are used to improve stroke volume and cardiac output, vasodilators (nitrates, hydralazine) are used to reduce the oxygen demand on the heart via preload and afterload reduction, and beta adrenergic blocking agents (propranolol) may be used to decrease myocardial oxygen consumption by reducing heart rate and blocking excessive catecholamine stimulation of the diseased heart. Diuretic, steroid, antidysrhythmic, and anticoagulant agents may also be used to treat or control complications associated with DC. The only surgical intervention for DC is heart transplant.

The treatment for HC is focused on improving ventricular filling and avoiding situations that may impair venous return or increase afterload. Beta adrenergic blocking agents and calcium channel blocking agents (verapamil, nifedipine) may be used to reduce left ventricular outflow obstruction and angina. Antidysrhythmic agents such as amiodarone can be used to treat dysrhythmias that compromise cardiac output. Positive inotropic and vasodilating agents are contraindicated, because they are capable of increasing the outflow gradient. Thus the development of heart failure is a difficult problem to treat. Conditions that may aggravate obstructive hypertrophic cardiomyopathy should be avoided, including strenuous exercise, stressful situations, and the Valsalva maneuver, since syncope or sudden death may result. Endocarditis prophylaxis is also prescribed. When medical therapy fails, surgical intervention

Table 1-13 Diagnostic findings associated with cardiomyopathies

Dilated Cardiomyopathy

Chest x-ray	Cardiomegaly, pulmonary venous congestion
ECG	Sinus tachycardia, dysrhythmias and conduction disturbances, abnormal Q waves without infarction; low voltage QRS; flat or inverted T waves
Echocardiography	Dilated ventricles; decreased wall motion; global hypokinesia; abnormal septal contractility; displacement of the mitral valve toward posterior wall of left ventricle; presence of thrombus; pericardial effusion may be present
Cardiac catheterization	Left ventricular enlargement, decreased contractility of ventricles; mitral regurgitation; elevated left ventricular end diastolic, left atrial, and wedge pressures

Hypertrophic Cardiomyopathy

Chest x-ray	Can demonstrate normal cardiac features or enlarged left atrium or ventricle
ECG	Abnormal P waves suggestive of atrial enlargement; ST segment and T wave abnormalities; left ventricular hypertrophy; increased QRS voltage in midprecordial leads; abnormal Q waves in leads II, III, aVF and V_4-V_6; left axis deviation; dysrhythmias

Echocardiography	Asymmetrical septal hypertrophy (ratio of septal wall thickness to posterior left ventricular wall is >1.5); abnormal septal motion; displacement of the mitral valve toward the septum; abnormal systolic anterior movement of the anterior mitral valve leaflet; decreased systolic ventricular volume
Cardiac catheterization	Outflow tract gradient may be present at rest or when provoked; ventricular shape may be distorted (hourglass configuration) because of large papillary muscles

Restrictive Cardiomyopathy

Chest x-ray	Cardiomegaly; pulmonary congestion
ECG	Low QRS voltage; P wave changes with atrial enlargement; dysrhythmias; conduction disturbances; left and right ventricular hypertrophy; right axis deviation
Echocardiography	Increased thickening of left ventricular wall; pericardial effusion; thrombus; atrial dilatation; normal systolic function; small or normal left ventricular cavity
Cardiac catheterization	Differentiates RC from constrictive pericarditis; elevated filling pressures (left greater than right); thickened endocardium and decreased ventricular size

may be employed. Select patients can benefit from partial septal resections.

Treatment for RC includes pharmacologic agents such as furosemide, digoxin, and prazosin to control heart failure and anticoagulant agents to reduce embolization. Corticosteroids and immunosuppressants have limited success in the treatment of RC. Pericardioperitoneal shunts may relieve tamponade, while surgical resection of thickened endocardial tissue may relieve symptoms. A pacemaker may be needed in patients who develop heart block.

Priorities of care are similar to those in patients with congestive heart failure. Generally, care includes assessment of cardiac output, evaluation of patient response to therapy, monitoring of ECG for dysrhythmia development, reduction of myocardial workload (e.g., bedrest, anxiety reduction), and education of the patient and family about the disease, medications, activity level and precautions to be taken against infective endocarditis.

Clinical Alert

Nitrates should not be given for chest discomfort or pain in patients with HC, since these agents can intensify the outflow tract gradient.

Pericarditis

Overview

Pericarditis is an inflammation of the fibroserous sac that encloses the heart and root of the great vessels. It can be the primary problem or a complication of another disease process. Common causes of pericarditis include myocardial infarction, infection, diseases of connective tissue, cardiac surgery, trauma, neoplasm, radiation exposure, drugs (procainamide, hydralazine, phenytoin), and uremia. Acute pericarditis associated with a myocardial infarction usually occurs within 2 to 3 days of the infarction. Late onset of pericarditis (3 to 6 weeks after myocardial infarction) is known as Dressler's syndrome.

Pericarditis with effusion can lead to cardiac tamponade (see the box headed "Cardiac Tamponade," on p. 234). This life-threatening condition is a result of rapid fluid accumulation in the pericardium that prevents adequate diastolic filling and reduces stroke volume. Compensatory mechanisms of tachycardia and increased vascular resistance fail to maintain cardiac output. Constrictive pericarditis may develop as a result of acute pericarditis and compromise cardiac output. Signs and symptoms of right-sided heart failure are produced.

Major Subjective/Objective Data

Chest pain that is aggravated by deep inspiration and relieved when the patient sits up and leans forward is characteristic of acute pericarditis. A pericardial friction rub, which may be intermittent and last for hours or days, is the predominant physical finding. The patient may also experience dyspnea and orthopnea if pericardial effusion develops. Faint heart sounds, decreased cardiac output, and hypotension may be indicative of cardiac tamponade, a life-threatening event (see the box on p. 234).

Diagnostic Tests

Diagnosis of pericarditis is difficult because abnormal findings demonstrated on ECG, x-ray, and echocardiography are not specific to this clinical disorder. The chest x-ray and echocardiogram are usually normal in patients with acute pericarditis without effusion. The ECG may reveal ST elevation in all leads (except aVR and V_1) occurring over several days, then returning to normal, followed by T wave inversion. If effusion is present, the echocardiogram may be helpful in determining its size and location. An enlarged cardiac silhouette may be noted on a chest x-ray. Refer to Chapter 2 for additional information on cardiovascular diagnostic tests.

Treatment

Treatment depends on the type of pericarditis and on symptomatology. Analgesic and antiinflammatory agents (usually aspirin, indomethacin, or ibuprofen) are prescribed to reduce pain. Cardiac tamponade should not be confused with other causes of increased venous pressure (congestive heart failure), since the treatment is not the same. Administration of diuretics or other treatments performed in an attempt to reduce intravascular volume in patients with tamponade may further reduce cardiac output. Recurrent pericarditis may be treated with steroids; however, steroid-induced complications may occur. Surgical intervention (pericardiectomy) may be needed in recurrent pericarditis and is usually the treatment for constrictive pericarditis.

Priorities of care include assessment of hemodynamic parameters, evaluation of patient response to therapy, detection of tamponade, and education of the patient and family regarding the nature of the disease, medications, and signs and symptoms of recurrent pericarditis (fever, cough, and pain).

Clinical Alert

Assess for signs and symptoms of cardiac tamponade (see the box on p. 234). Should cardiac tamponade develop, an emergency pericardiocentesis or pericardiectomy may be necessary.

Endocarditis

Overview

Infective endocarditis is a condition that affects the endothelial lining of the heart and is caused by circulating microbes. Vegetations, which may increase in size and potentially obstruct valvular openings, characterize this disorder. A leading cause of death is congestive heart failure secondary to acute aortic regurgitation. Emboli may develop and cause multiple organ infarcts and mycotic aneurysms. Patients with preexisting heart disease, such as mitral valve prolapse and valve disease, are at risk for infective endocarditis. However, patients with no known heart disease, such as IV drug users, can also develop endocarditis.

Streptococci and staphylococci cause the majority of infective endocarditis cases. Highly virulent organisms can produce extensive damage to the chordae tendineae, papillary muscle, conduction system, and valves. Although the aortic and mitral valves are most commonly affected, the tricuspid valve is frequently involved in IV drug users. Entry of the organism into the bloodstream can occur after dental procedures and surgeries, with infectious conditions, and with use of invasive equipment.

Complications of infective endocarditis include heart failure (secondary to valvular damage), embolization, and mycotic aneurysms. Embolization may occur several weeks or months after the valvular infectious process has been eradicated. Common sites of embolization include kidneys, spleen, coronary vessels, and brain. Mycotic aneurysms may not manifest for months or years after the infectious process has been eradicated. They can develop in any artery during the active phase of the infection. However, patients may remain asymptomatic until the aneurysm starts to leak or ruptures.

Major Subjective/Objective Data

The onset and progress of infective endocarditis are variable and can range from a flu-like illness to an acute life-threatening disease process. Clinical manifestations of infective endocarditis are a result of systemic infection, intravascular lesions, and immunologic reactions. Symptoms suggestive of systemic infection include general malaise, headache, fatigue, chills, fever, weight loss, and night sweats. Pain in the chest, abdomen, or flank area may be manifestations of embolization and infarction. Immunologic reactions and intravascular lesions may account for the following peripheral signs: petechiae, Janeway lesions, Osler's nodes, and splinter and retinal hemorrhages. Focal neurologic signs may be caused by embolization to the central nervous system. Murmurs are frequently present in patients with endocarditis. Symptoms can worsen and cardiac failure may develop (or worsen) as a result of valvular damage.

Diagnostic Tests

Diagnosis of infective endocarditis can be delayed in many cases because of its indolent course or its initial misleading presentation. Diagnosis is based on clinical findings and blood culture results. Infective endocarditis should be suspected in patients who have fever, murmur, and anemia. The diagnostic tests performed when a patient is suspected of having endocarditis are listed in Table 1-14. Refer to Chapter 2 for additional information on cardiovascular diagnostic tests.

Treatment

Because of the seriousness of infective endocarditis, antibiotic prophylaxis is required in patients at high risk who are undergoing dental or surgical procedures and instrumentation (Table 1-15).

Intravenous antibiotic therapy is the treatment for infective endocarditis; it is prescribed for 2 to 6 weeks or longer, depending on the organism and the patient's response. Without treatment, endocarditis is fatal. Relapses and reinfections can occur. Anticoagulant therapy with heparin is generally avoided in patients with endocarditis. Surgery may be required to replace infected or damaged valves.

The care of patients with endocarditis includes careful and accurate administration of antibiotics; management of IV sites, in-

Table 1-14   Diagnostic tests for endocarditis

Test	Findings
Blood culture	Isolation of an organism, although it may be negative
Hematology	Increase in sedimentation rate, decrease in serum complement level, and anemia may be present
Chest x-ray	May provide evidence of heart failure and pulmonary infiltrates, suggesting septic emboli
ECG	May indicate extension of the infection into myocardium, if new conduction disturbances develop
Echocardiography	May demonstrate valvular vegetations if greater than 3 to 4 mm in size; is used to monitor progress of cardiac function and size of vegetations; a false negative test is possible because not all valve leaflets can be visualized
Cardiac catheterization	Used to evaluate ventricular and valvular function; useful for evaluating patients for possible surgical intervention

cluding early detection of signs of local infection; and careful monitoring of the patient's response to therapy and any adverse effects of antibiotic therapy. In addition, the patient should be carefully evaluated for complications of heart failure and embolization. Educating the high-risk patient about endocarditis, proper oral and dental hygiene, compliance with antibiotic prophylaxis, and signs and symptoms of relapse is also necessary.

Valvular Dysfunction

Overview

Cardiac valves allow for the unidirectional flow of blood through the heart. If a valve does not open properly, it is stenotic and the forward flow of blood is obstructed. This causes increased pressure proximal to the obstruction and the potential for decreased flow distally. The primary response of the heart to the increased pressure

Table 1-15   **Endocarditis prophylaxis**
I. Recommended standard prophylactic regimen for
dental, oral, or upper respiratory tract procedures in patients
who are at risk*

Drug	Dosing Regimen†
Standard Regimen	
Amoxicillin	3.0 g orally 1 h before procedure; then 1.5 g 6 h after initial dose
Amoxicillin/Penicillin-Allergic Patients	
Erythromycin	Erythromycin ethylsuccinate, 800 mg, or erythromycin stearate, 1.0 g, orally 2 h
or	before procedure; then half the dose 6 h after initial dose
Clindamycin	300 mg orally 1 h before procedure and 150 mg 6 h after initial dose

From Prevention of Bacterial Endocarditis, 1991, American Heart Association.
*Includes those with prosthetic heart valves and other high-risk patients.
†Initial pediatric doses are as follows: amoxicillin, 50 mg/kg; erythromycin ethylsuccinate or erythromycin stearate, 20 mg/kg; and clindamycin, 10 mg/kg. Follow-up doses should be one half the initial dose. Total pediatric dose should not exceed total adult dose. The following weight ranges may also be used for the initial pediatric dose of amoxicillin: <15 kg, 750 mg; 15 to 30 kg, 1500 mg; and >30 kg, 3000 mg (full adult dose).

Continued.

is hypertrophy or increased muscle mass, which is beneficial in compensating for the obstruction but costly in terms of myocardial oxygen consumption.

When a valve does not close properly, blood leaks or regurgitates from one area back into another. The regurgitant volume results in dilatation or increased chamber size. The dilatation is an effective compensatory mechanism for a time, but eventually it increases myocardial oxygen consumption, potentially leading to ventricular failure. In addition, the enlarged chamber may compress adjacent structures; for example, an enlarged left atrium may compress the esophagus, resulting in dysphagia.

Most acquired valve disease affects the mitral and aortic valves. Common causes of valvular dysfunction include rheumatic endocarditis, nonrheumatic endocarditis, calcification, papillary muscle dysfunction, chordae rupture, mitral valve prolapse, myxomatous

Table 1-15   Endocarditis prophylaxis—cont'd
II. Alternate prophylactic regimens for dental, oral, or upper respiratory tract procedures in patients who are at risk

Drug	Dosing Regimen*
Patients Unable to Take Oral Medications	
Ampicillin	Intravenous or intramuscular administration of ampicillin, 2.0 g, 30 min before procedure; then intravenous or intramuscular administration of ampicillin, 1.0 g, or oral administration of amoxicillin, 1.5 g, 6 h after initial dose
Ampicillin/Amoxicillin/Penicillin-Allergic Patients Unable to Take Oral Medications	
Clindamycin	Intravenous administration of 300 mg 30 min before procedure and an intravenous or oral administration of 150 mg 6 h after initial dose
Patients Considered High Risk and Not Candidates for Standard Regimen	
Ampicillin, gentamicin, and amoxicillin	Intravenous or intramuscular administration of ampicillin, 2.0 g, plus gentamicin, 1.5 mg/kg (not to exceed 80 mg), 30 min before procedure; followed by amoxicillin, 1.5 g, orally 6 h after initial dose; alternatively, the parenteral regimen may be repeated 8 h after initial dose
Ampicillin/Amoxicillin/Penicillin-Allergic Patients Considered High Risk	
Vancomycin	Intravenous administration of 1.0 g over 1 h, starting 1 h before procedure; no repeated dose necessary

From Prevention of Bacterial Endocarditis, 1991, American Heart Association.
*Initial pediatric doses are as follows: ampicillin, 50 mg/kg; clindamycin, 10 mg/kg; gentamicin, 2.0 mg/kg; and vancomycin, 20 mg/kg. Follow-up doses should be one half the initial dose. Total pediatric dose should not exceed total adult dose. No initial dose is recommended in this table for amoxicillin (25 mg/kg is the follow-up dose).

⋏Table 1-15   Endocarditis prophylaxis—cont'd
III. Regimens for genitourinary/gastrointestinal procedures

Drug	Dosage Regimen*
Standard Regimen	
Ampicillin, gentamicin, and amoxicillin	Intravenous or intramuscular administration of ampicillin, 2.0 g, plus gentamicin, 1.5 mg/kg (not to exceed 80 mg), 30 min before procedure; followed by amoxicillin, 1.5 g, orally 6 h after initial dose; alternatively, the parenteral regimen may be repeated once 8 h after initial dose
Ampicillin/Amoxicillin/Penicillin-Allergic Patient Regimen	
Vancomycin and gentamicin	Intravenous administration of vancomycin, 1.0 g, over 1 h plus intravenous or intramuscular administration of gentamicin, 1.5 mg/kg (not to exceed 80 mg), 1 h before procedure; may be repeated once 8 h after initial dose
Alternate Low-Risk Patient Regimen	
Amoxicillin	3.0 g orally 1 h before procedure; then 1.5 g 6 h after initial dose

From Prevention of Bacterial Endocarditis, 1991, American Heart Association.
*Initial pediatric doses are as follows: ampicillin, 50 mg/kg; amoxicillin, 50 mg/kg; gentamicin, 2.0 mg/kg; and vancomycin, 20 mg/kg. Follow-up doses should be half the initial dose. Total pediatric dose should not exceed total adult dose.

Table 1-16 Clinical manifestations of mitral and aortic valve disease

Mitral stenosis	Dyspnea, orthopnea, PND, palpitations, fatigue, hemoptysis, symptoms of right ventricular failure (late), decreased pulse pressure, loud S_1, diastolic murmur, opening snap
Mitral insufficiency (mitral regurgitation)	Dyspnea, fatigue, symptoms of right ventricular failure (late), pansystolic murmur that radiates to axilla, S_3, soft S_1, widely split S_2, S_4 (acute mitral insufficiency)
Mitral valve prolapse	Chest pain atypical for angina; palpitations; symptoms of left ventricular failure due to mitral regurgitation; systolic click; skeletal abnormalities, such as scoliosis or pectus excavatum
Aortic stenosis	Angina, dyspnea and other indications of ventricular dysfunction, syncope, plateau pulse, systolic crescendo-decrescendo murmur, ejection click, left ventricular heave or lift, sustained PMI, S_4, S_3
Aortic insufficiency (aortic regurgitation)	Dyspnea, palpitations, symptoms of left ventricular failure, diastolic decrescendo murmur, wide pulse pressure, hyperdynamic pulse (water-hammer pulse, Corrigan's pulse), head bobbing (deMusset's sign), capillary pulsations (Quincke's sign), systolic pulsations of uvula (Müller's sign), systolic murmur over femoral artery when compressed proximally, diastolic murmur when compressed distally (Duroziez's sign), S_3

PND, paroxysmal nocturnal dyspnea. PMI, point of maximal impulse.

degeneration, bicuspid valve (aortic stenosis), and connective tissue disease, such as Marfan's syndrome.

Major Subjective/Objective Data

Clinical manifestations of mitral and aortic valve disease are presented in Table 1-16. Any combination of these manifestations may be present.

Diagnostic Tests

The ECG provides information about the effects produced by valvular dysfunction, that is, dysrhythmias, chamber enlargement, axis deviation, and conduction delays. The chest x-ray may show evidence of pulmonary congestion, cardiac enlargement, calcification of a valve, or aortic dilatation—again, all effects produced by valvular dysfunction. More helpful in diagnosing the extent of valvular dysfunction are the echocardiogram and cardiac catheterization. Echocardiography provides a noninvasive, risk-free means of assessing valve function and determining chamber size. Via cardiac catheterization, valve orifice size can be calculated, pressure gradients across narrowed valves measured, the amount of regurgitant flow estimated, and ventricular function evaluated. See Table 1-17 for diagnostic findings associated with mitral and aortic valve disease. Refer to Chapter 2 for additional information on diagnostic tests.

Treatment

Valvular dysfunction is progressive. Management may be medical, surgical, or a combination. The medical approach is appropriate for the problems identified in Table 1-18. Percutaneous balloon valvuloplasty is becoming a more frequent nonsurgical alternative for the patient with critical valvular stenosis. The procedure is performed in a cardiac catheterization laboratory. Nursing care is similar to that for percutaneous transluminal coronary angioplasty (PTCA), discussed in Chapter 5.

Surgically, the valve may be repaired (commissurotomy, valvuloplasty) or totally replaced. Prosthetic valves may be either mechanical or bioprosthetic (tissue). The major advantage of a mechanical valve is durability; the major disadvantage is thrombogenicity, which necessitates anticoagulation with its inherent risks. Bioprosthetics are less thrombogenic but not as durable as mechanical valves. The type of valve prosthesis to be used, along with the

Table 1-17   Possible diagnostic findings of mitral and aortic valve disease

Mitral Stenosis

ECG
: May be normal; broad notched P wave (P-mitrale) predominant in lead II; atrial fibrillation common; if pulmonary hypertension and RV hypertrophy are present, right axis deviation, tall R waves in V_1, V_2

Chest x-ray
: Double density at right heart border, straightening of left heart border, calcification at valve area, altered pulmonary venous pattern, enlarged RV

Echocardiography
: Thickened mitral leaflets, abnormal movement of mitral leaflets, enlarged LA, decreased size of valve orifice, vegetations on leaflets

Cardiac catheterization
: Gradient across mitral valve

Mitral Insufficiency

ECG
: May be normal; atrial fibrillation; LA enlargement; LV hypertrophy

Chest x-ray
: May be normal; enlarged cardiac silhouette; pulmonary venous congestion

Echocardiography
: Large LV and LA; hyperdynamic LV motion

Cardiac catheterization
: LV angiogram demonstrates reflux of contrast through mitral valve into LA

Mitral Valve Prolapse

ECG
: May be normal; ST segment depression, T wave inversion; QT prolongation; atrial and ventricular tachydysrhythmias; bradydysrhythmias

Chest x-ray	Usually normal; skeletal abnormalities may be visualized
Echocardiography	Abnormal movement of mitral valve
Cardiac catheterization	If mitral insufficiency present, LV angiogram demonstrates reflux of contrast through mitral valve into LA

Aortic Stenosis

ECG	LV hypertrophy, ST and T wave changes; AV block and BBB
Chest x-ray	Calcified aortic valve; poststenotic aortic root dilatation; if heart failure, enlarged cardiac silhouette, pulmonary congestion
Echocardiography	Thickened, calcified aortic valve cusps; decreased mobility of valve; LV hypertrophy; vegetations on valve leaflets
Cardiac catheterization	Gradient across valve; fluoroscopy demonstrates valve calcification

Aortic Insufficiency

ECG	LV hypertrophy
Chest x-ray	Enlarged cardiac silhouette
Echocardiography	Increased LV and aortic size; fluttering of anterior mitral leaflet
Cardiac catheterization	Aortic root injection demonstrates reflux of contrast from aorta into LV

RV, right ventricle. LV, left ventricle. LA, left atrium. AV, atrioventricular. BBB, bundle branch block.

Table 1-18   Medical therapy for valvular dysfunction

Problem	Treatment
Atrial fibrillation with uncontrolled ventricular response	Digitalis
Embolic phenomena caused by atrial fibrillation	Warfarin
Development of signs and symptoms of heart failure	Digitalis, diuretics, salt restriction, afterload reduction
Endocarditis	Antibiotics
Narrowed valve orifice	Percutaneous balloon valvuloplasty

proper timing of the operation, must be carefully considered with each patient to obtain maximum results.

Once a valve is repaired or replaced, medical management must continue to identify and treat the following potential problems: anemia resulting from intravascular hemolysis, valve dysfunction, valve infection, thromboembolism, and bleeding related to anticoagulation.

The patient with valvular dysfunction, whether treated medically or surgically, may experience problems such as valve infection; decreased cardiac output related to dysrhythmias or ventricular dysfunction; bleeding associated with anticoagulation; discomfort from chest pain, shortness of breath, or palpitations; and a limited tolerance of activity because of poor cardiac function. Priorities of care include careful assessment for early identification of these problems, evaluation of response to therapy, and identification of teaching needs. Information about medications, importance of spacing activities, significance of pain and other symptoms, use of relaxation techniques, and endocarditis prophylaxis (see Table 1-15) should be a part of the teaching plan for the patient with valvular dysfunction.

Congenital Heart Disease

Overview

Congenital heart disease refers to cardiac defects present at birth. Clinical manifestations of a heart defect may be present at birth or

✕ Table 1-19   Common congenital heart defects

Defect	Description
Acyanotic With Shunt	
Atrial septal defect (ASD)	Opening in interatrial septum allows communication between left atrium and right atrium
Ventricular septal defect (VSD)	Opening in interventricular septum allows communication between left ventricle and right ventricle
Patent ductus arteriosus (PDA)	Fetal vessel, ductus arteriosus, between the aorta and pulmonary artery fails to close
Acyanotic Without Shunt (Obstructive)	
Aortic stenosis (AS)	Aortic valve impedes flow from left ventricle to aorta
Coarctation	Obstruction in aorta (usually distal to left subclavian) impedes flow to mesentery and lower extremities
Pulmonic stenosis (PS)	Pulmonary valve or small pulmonary artery impedes flow from right ventricle into pulmonary artery
Cyanotic	
Tetralogy of Fallot	Defects include VSD, PS, overriding aorta (overrides VSD), and right ventricular hypertrophy
Transposition of the great vessels (TGV)	Aorta (with the coronary arteries) exits from right ventricle, pulmonary artery exits from left ventricle, systemic and pulmonary circuits are parallel rather than serial

Continued.

Table 1-19   Common congenital heart defects—cont'd

Defect	Description
Truncus arteriosus	One large vessel leaves the heart; it receives blood from both the right and left ventricles
Tricuspid atresia	Lack of tricuspid valve
Total anomalous pulmonary venous return (TAPVR)	Pulmonary veins ultimately empty into the right atrium rather than the left atrium

may not be apparent for months or years. The incidence of congenital heart disease, excluding bicuspid aortic valve, is approximately 0.8% of live births. Although a specific cause cannot be identified 90% of the time, increased risk of a heart defect is associated with advanced maternal age, exposure to radiation, infectious disease such as rubella during pregnancy, and certain genetic factors.

Congenital heart defects can be classified as acyanotic or cyanotic (Table 1-19). Acyanotic defects may be obstructive without a shunt (aortic stenosis) or nonobstructive with a left to right shunt, where oxygenated blood from the left side of the circulation is recirculated to the lungs (atrial septal defect). With an obstructive lesion, increased afterload for the ventricle is of concern; with a left to right shunt major concerns are pulmonary flooding and right ventricular overload. Ultimately, pulmonary hypertension, caused by pulmonary flooding, can result in right ventricular failure and reversal of the shunt.

Cyanotic defects are those with a right to left shunt, that is, desaturated blood from the right side of the heart bypasses the lungs and is pumped out of the aorta. Thus desaturated blood reaches the systemic circulation. The end result is chronic hypoxemia, which is responsible for many of the signs and symptoms seen with a cyanotic lesion.

Major Subjective/Objective Data

Because of improved surgical techniques, more children with congenital heart disease survive to become adults. Complete repair of a defect at an early age may result in a normal life without symptoms. Some patients, however, will have signs and symptoms as a result of incomplete repair, residual defects, or complications from surgery.

Manifestations of acyanotic lesions with a shunt include frequent upper respiratory infections, respiratory distress, slow growth, and supraventricular dysrhythmias; ultimately, evidence of right ventricular failure from pulmonary hypertension with potential reversal of shunt and left ventricular failure is seen. Ventricular failure is the major manifestation of acyanotic lesions without a shunt. Coarctation is suggested by hypertension, delayed femoral pulse, the upper body being larger in proportion to the lower body, claudication, headaches, and leg fatigue.

Cyanotic defects are associated with the following: bluish color of warm mucous membranes (central cyanosis), clubbing of digits, squatting, evidence of thromboembolic events (cerebrovascular accident, loss of femoral pulse), cyanotic attacks (hyperpnea, cyanosis, lightheadedness, or syncope), or evidence of brain abscess (fever, neurologic deficit).

See Table 1-20 for auscultatory findings associated with congenital heart defects.

Diagnostic Tests

The ECG may assist in diagnosing a congenital heart defect or in identifying the effects of the defect. ECG findings may include axis deviation, chamber enlargement, conduction defects, and dysrhythmias. The chest x-ray may demonstrate enlarged chambers and vessels, pulmonary congestion, and abnormal anatomy (such as a right aortic arch). Echocardiography is helpful in determining the size of chambers, movement of valves, and continuity of septum and in identifying other anatomic structures. Cardiac catheterization is the most definitive diagnostic test. It provides information about the anatomy of the heart and great vessels and aids in assessment of ventricular function. In addition, cardiac catheterization provides access for palliative procedures, such as balloon septostomy. Refer to Chapter 2 for additional information on diagnostic tests.

Treatment

Medical treatment of congenital heart disease consists primarily of the following: control of heart failure with digitalis and diuretics,

Table 1-20 Auscultatory findings associated with congenital heart defects

Defect	Findings
ASD	Systolic flow murmur across pulmonic valve; diastolic flow murmur across tricuspid valve; wide, fixed split of S_2
VSD	Pansystolic murmur at LSB; if pulmonary hypertension exists, pulmonic ejection murmur; pulmonic ejection click; diastolic decrescendo murmur of pulmonary insufficiency; pansystolic murmur of tricuspid insufficiency may occur
PDA	Continuous, machinery murmur LUSB; if pulmonary hypertension exists, see VSD
AS	Systolic crescendo-decrescendo ejection murmur RUSB with radiation to carotids and down LSB to apex, ejection click, single or paradoxical splitting of S_2, S_4 with severe obstruction
PS	Pulmonic ejection murmur, wide split of S_2, soft or absent P_2, S_4 with severe obstruction
Coarctation	Late systolic or continuous murmur, S_4
Tetralogy of Fallot	Pulmonic ejection murmur, soft to absent P_2, no murmur across VSD resulting from equalization of ventricular pressures
Transposition of great vessels	No murmurs may be audible
Truncus arteriosus	Systolic murmur at LSB, continuous murmur over both lung fields, diastolic murmur resulting from truncal insufficiency
Tricuspid atresia	No murmur or systolic murmur at LSB, gallop rhythm
Total anomalous pulmonary venous return	Systolic murmur at LSB, prominent S_3, S_4, fixed split of S_2

ASD, atrial septal defect. VSD, ventricular septal defect. PDA, patent ductus arteriosus. AS, aortic stenosis. PS, pulmonic stenosis. LSB, left sternal border. LUSB, left upper sternal border. RUSB, right upper sternal border.

attempts to close a PDA with indomethacin, attempts to keep the ductus arteriosus open with prostaglandins, and attempts to improve arterial saturation with balloon septostomy. Surgical intervention when indicated is tailored to the specific defect(s) present. Total correction, however, is not always possible.

Priorities of care include careful assessment for potential problems (i.e., worsening cyanosis, dysrhythmias, evidence of heart failure, thromboembolic events, and infection). Teaching the patient and family concerning the defect, complications, treatment, and life-style adjustments must also be considered. See Chapter 6 for detailed information on patient and family teaching.

Hypertension

Overview

Hypertension is a major health problem in the United States. It is a leading cause of heart attacks and strokes. Hypertension is defined by the American Heart Association as a blood pressure above 140/90. National Instiues of Health defines hypertension as systolic pressure 140 or greater and/or diastolic pressure 90 or greater. There is no identifiable cause for elevated blood pressure in 90% to 95% of patients with the condition, and therefore they will be diagnosed as having primary or essential hypertension. If a cause can be determined, the term secondary hypertension is used. Causes of secondary hypertension can be found in Table 1-21.

Table 1-21   Causes of secondary hypertension

Renal disease	Acute glomerulonephritis, renal tumors, chronic pyelonephritis, renovascular hypertension
Endocrine disorders	Primary aldosteronism, Cushing's syndrome, pheochromocytoma, hyperparathyroidism
Vascular Disorders	Coarctation
Pregnancy-related disorders	Preeclampsia, eclampsia
Drug-related disorders	Birth control pills, steroids, cyclosporine

Table 1-22   **Characteristics of a hypertensive crisis**

Diastolic blood pressure	Usually >140 mm Hg
Funduscopic examination	Hemorrhages, exudates, papill-edema
Neurologic	Headache, confusion, stupor, seizures, visual deficits, coma
Cardiac	Evidence of congestive failure, pulmonary edema, myocardial infarction
Renal	Oliguria, azotemia
Gastrointestinal	Nausea, vomiting

A small group of patients with hypertension will develop rapid progression of their disease, which will result in a hypertensive crisis. The blood pressure is characteristically extremely high, and if not aggressively treated, irreversible tissue damage and death will occur. There is no specific level of blood pressure that defines hypertensive crisis. Rather the rate and degree of change in pressure plus resultant end organ damage are significant. Characteristics of a hypertensive crisis can be found in Table 1-22.

Systemic arterial blood pressure is determined by cardiac output and vascular resistance. An alteration of flow in the vascular compartment (increased or decreased ventricular function, increased or decreased intravascular volume) or an alteration in vascular resistance (vasoconstriction/vasodilatation) will influence blood pressure. With hypertension, usually there is a component of increased volume or vasoconstriction. Whether primary or secondary hypertension, the eventual effect of the elevated pressure is vascular injury and end organ damage. In addition, the atherosclerotic process is accelerated. Organs most commonly affected are the brain/eye, heart, kidneys, and blood vessels (Table 1-23).

Major Subjective/Objective Data

The majority of patients with hypertension are asymptomatic for many years. Symptoms that do occur can be related to the effect of high blood pressure on target organs or a secondary cause of hypertension. Vague discomfort, fatigue, headache, epistaxis, and dizziness may be early indicators of hypertension. As the disease

Table 1-23   Complications of hypertension

Target Organ	Complication
Brain/eye	Intracerebral hemorrhage, thrombotic stroke, encephalopathy, fundal hemorrhages, exudates, papilledema
Heart	Congestive failure, ventricular hypertrophy, angina, myocardial infarction, sudden death
Kidney	Nephrosclerosis, renal artery stenosis
Peripheral vessels	Aortic dissection, diffuse atherosclerosis

progresses, the patient may experience a throbbing suboccipital headache, confusion, visual loss, focal deficits, and coma. Symptoms of heart failure, such as dyspnea, may be present. The patient may experience angina or myocardial infarction. If the kidneys are affected, hematuria or nocturia may be noticed. Vascular involvement may be suggested by the "tearing" pain of aortic dissection or claudication and rest pain caused by accelerated peripheral vascular disease. Paroxysmal sweating, palpitations, flushing, and headache may be associated with pheochromocytoma (adrenal tumor).

Objective data include documentation of elevated blood pressure by accurately taking three resting measurements at 3- to 5-minute intervals (see the box on p. 138). Use of nicotine, caffeine, or other stimulants that may elevate the blood pressure should be noted. Other objective findings are listed in Table 1-24.

Diagnostic Tests

The diagnosis of hypertension is made on the basis of three blood pressure measurements. Of utmost importance to the diagnosis is the accuracy of these measurements. Ideally, the patient is relaxed and sees the environment as nonthreatening. Diagnostic tests are useful to evaluate the effects of the elevated pressure on target organs and also to identify secondary forms of hypertension. See Table 1-25 for specific findings. Refer to Chapter 2 for additional information on diagnostic tests.

Treatment

The cornerstone of medical therapy is modification of risk factors: weight reduction, smoking cessation, stress reduction, regular aero-

Table 1-24   Objective findings associated with hypertension

Parameter	Finding	Possible Cause
Cardiac	LV heave (5ICS at MCL), S_4, PMI at AAL, S_3, crackles (if failure is present), pulsus alternans	LV hypertrophy, congestive failure
Vascular	Diminished/absent pulses	Accelerated PVOD
	Radial/femoral pulse lag, hypertension in arms, normal to low pressure in legs	Coarctation
Neurologic	Positive Babinski sign, hemiparesis, ataxia, confusion, cognitive changes	Cerebral ischemia, cerebral infarct
Eye	Hemorrhage, exudates, arteriovenous nicking, papilledema	Vascular damage to ocular vessels
Renal	Renal artery bruit	Renal artery stenosis
	Edema	Renal disease
Other	Episodic hypertension, orthostatic hypotension	Pheochromocytoma

LV, left ventricle. ICS, intercostal space. MCL, midclavicular line. PMI, point of maximal impulse. AAL, anterior axillary line. PVOD, peripheral vascular occlusive disease.

Table 1-25   Diagnostic findings in the hypertensive patient

Test	Finding	Possible Etiology
Blood chemistry	Serum creatinine >1.3 mg/dl, BUN >20 mg/dl	Renal parenchymal disease
	RBC low	Hematuria
Urinalysis/urine culture	Specific gravity <1.010, proteinuria	Renal impairment
	Hematuria, granular or red cell casts	Glomerulonephritis
	Bacteria	Pyelonephritis
	VMA ↑ (24-hour urine)	Pheochromocytoma
	Cortisol or ACTH ↑ (24-hour urine)	Cushing's disease
ECG	Increased QRS voltage, ST-T wave changes, axis deviation	LV hypertrophy
Echocardiography	Increased LV wall thickness	LV hypertrophy
	Increased LV chamber size	LV dilatation
Chest x-ray	Enlarged cardiac silhouette	Enlarged LV
	Pulmonary congestion	Congestive failure
	Notching of aorta/ribs, dilated aortic root	Coarctation
	Widened aortic shadow	Aortic dissection

LV, left ventricle. VMA, vanillymandelic acid. ACTH, adrenocorticotropic hormone.

bic exercise, and reduction of sodium and alcohol intake. If these measures are not adequate to control blood pressure, medication may be added. Antihypertensive drugs increase the size of the vascular compartment and diuretics decrease blood volume; both effects potentially decrease blood pressure. Specific information about drugs can be found in Chapter 4.

Surgical treatment may be effective for some forms of secondary hypertension, since the cause can be identified. Renal artery bypass or renal artery angioplasty may be the treatment of choice for renal artery stenosis. Coarctation of the aorta can be repaired by removing the narrowed area and inserting a graft. If pheochromocytoma is the cause of hypertension, the tumor(s) can be surgically removed.

Because the patient is often asymptomatic or develops side effects after taking prescribed medications, the incidence of noncompliance with therapy is high. Patient teaching may positively affect compliance if it focuses on the effects of high blood pressure, risk factor modification, the technique for blood pressure measurement and recording, medications (including the need for physician approval before taking over-the-counter medications), and the necessity of ongoing treatment despite a feeling of well-being. Also of importance is monitoring for complications of therapy, such as volume depletion resulting in dizziness; hypokalemia or hyperkalemia, which may precipitate dysrhythmias; and hypochloremia, which may result in metabolic alkalosis. Prompt adjustment of therapy will minimize the effect of these or other complications.

Clinical Alert

Hypertension is a "silent killer." The health care professional is in a key role not only to detect hypertension but to enhance compliance with therapy through patient teaching.

Peripheral Vascular Occlusive Disease (PVOD)

Overview

PVOD itself is seldom life threatening; however, a significant number of patients with PVOD also have atherosclerotic disease elsewhere, such as the coronary arteries, carotid arteries, and renal arteries. Thus these patients are at high risk for myocardial infarction, cerebrovascular accident, and renal failure.

The major cause of PVOD is arteriosclerosis obliterans, atherosclerotic involvement of medium- and large-sized vessels. Figure 1-5 shows the common sites of PVOD. Arteries of the lower extremities are the most commonly affected and incidence is highest in men and diabetic individuals. Because atherosclerosis is the underlying problem, the risk factors for PVOD are the same as those for coronary artery disease. Signs and symptoms of PVOD result from a decreased blood flow through narrowed vessels, which re-

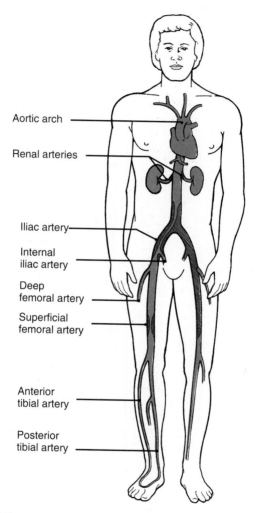

Figure 1-5
Common sites of peripheral vascular occlusive disease.

Table 1-26 Differential diagnosis of Raynaud's disease, thromboangiitis obliterans, and arteriosclerosis obliterans

	Raynaud's Disease	Thromboangiitis Obliterans	Arteriosclerosis Obliterans
Age of onset of symptoms	Adolescent to middle age	Young adult	Usually older than 50 years
Sex	Largely females	Largely males	Ratio of males/females, approximately 9:1; increased incidence in postmenopausal women
Upper versus lower extremity involvement	Upper	Upper and Lower	Lower
Concomitant venous pathologic condition	Absent	Frequent recurring superficial phlebitis	Absent

Calcification of involved arteries	Absent	Absent	Present in about 85% of cases
Audible bruits over major arteries	No	No	Frequent
Diminished or absent popliteal pulse(s)	No	Rare	Yes
Precipitated by cold or emotion	Yes	No	No
Associated risk factors			
Hyperlipidemia	Very rare	Rare	About 20% of patients
Diabetes mellitus	No known association	Absent	About 40% of younger patients
Cigarette smoking	No known association	>95% of patients	>95% of patients

From Guzzetta C, Dossey B: *Cardiovascular nursing: bodymind tapestry*, St Louis, 1984, Mosby.

sults in unmet demands of the tissues. Other less common causes of PVOD include thromboangiitis obliterans (Buerger's disease) and Raynaud's phenomenon (see Table 1-26). A cause of sudden peripheral occlusion is arterial embolism. The remainder of information presented here will relate to PVOD that results from its most common cause, atherosclerosis.

Major Subjective/Objective Data

Intermittent claudication, often the earliest indication of PVOD, is manifested by cramping, pain, or fatigue in muscles during exercise that is promptly relieved with rest. The calf muscle is often affected, but the discomfort may also occur in the thigh, hip, or buttocks.

As arterial blood supply decreases further, the patient may experience pain at rest. Rest pain typically occurs in the forefoot and is worse at night when the feet and legs are not dependent. When arterial blood supply is no longer adequate to meet even minimal demand at rest, ulceration and gangrene occur. Necrosis usually appears first on the distalmost portion of the toes. Arterial ulcers typically have a pale gray or yellowish base and are found on the toes, heel, and lateral aspect of the ankle.

Other signs consistent with PVOD include decreased or absent pulse; coolness of extremity; pale, shiny, dry skin; loss of hair distal to the occlusion; nail changes; dependent redness or rubor; increased pigmentation; and decreased capillary refill. See Table 2-7 for additional assessment information.

Diagnostic Tests

The arterial Doppler examination helps to identify the presence and location of arterial occlusion by determining segmental leg pressures, analogue wave tracings, and the ankle/arm index. With intermittent claudication, the ankle/arm index is usually 0.45 to 0.75; an index of <0.25 is consistent with severe ischemia.

Before surgery, arteriography is generally necessary to specifically identify the location and extent of the lesion and also to evaluate distal anatomy. Refer to Chapter 2 for additional information on diagnostic tests.

Treatment

Medical therapy for PVOD consists of exercise to the point of pain, discontinuation of smoking, avoidance of drugs that decrease peripheral flow (such as beta blockers), protection of extremities from extreme temperatures and trauma, prompt care of trauma or minor infections, control of risk factors, use of vasodilators (controversial) and hemorrheologic agents, balloon angioplasty, laser therapy, or atherectomy.

If symptoms continue or viability of tissue is of concern, surgical intervention becomes necessary. Increased blood flow may be provided by laser surgery or revascularization (see Table 5-3). Sympathectomy—the interruption of lumbar sympathetic ganglia, which results in permanent vasodilation primarily in skin vessels —is another surgical technique that may improve arterial flow to the skin but will not help pain at rest or claudication. If measures to improve arterial flow are unsuccessful and tissue is necrotic, amputation may be necessary.

For the patient with PVOD, education about risk factor modification and good foot care is essential. See Chapter 5 for a discussion of care after peripheral vascular surgery.

Aneurysms

Overview

An aneurysm is a weakness in a vessel resulting in a dilated area or a separation of the layers that make up the wall of the vessel. Aneurysms may be congenital or acquired as a result of syphilis, trauma, or atherosclerosis. True aneurysms, involving the wall of the vessel, may be saccular (localized outpouching), fusiform (circumferential dilatation), or dissecting (separation of wall layers) (see Figure 1-6). A false aneurysm results from a tear in the arterial wall, which allows a hematoma to form in the perivascular tissue. Although aneurysms may occur in any vessel, the most common locations are the thoracic aorta and abdominal aorta. Abdominal aneurysms most often occur distal to the renal arteries and are confined to the abdominal aorta. Patients with aneurysms often have significant atherosclerotic disease elsewhere, thus they are at risk for cardiac and neurologic events as well as renal dysfunction.

Major Subjective/Objective Data

Signs and symptoms of an aneurysm result from rupture of the aneurysm, compression on adjacent structures, embolization, or arterial occlusion. Most patients with aneurysms are asymptomatic until the aneurysm begins to expand, dissect, or leak. Pain is the most

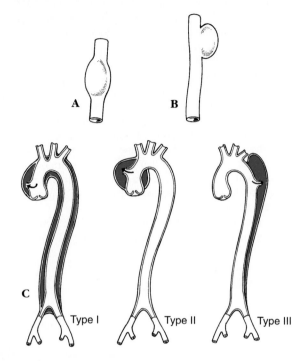

Figure 1-6
Types of aneurysms. **A,** Fusiform; **B,** saccular; **C,** dissecting.

common symptom and is related directly to the expansion of the vessel or to hypoperfusion of an organ or extremity. Refer to the box on p. 57 for common signs and symptoms of aneurysms.

Diagnostic Tests

Radiography can be helpful in diagnosing an aneurysm. A mediastinal mass on a chest film may be a thoracic aneurysm, while widening of the mediastinum may be seen with a dissection. Calcification in the wall of the aorta on an abdominal film is highly suggestive of an abdominal aneurysm. Ultrasound, CT scans, and MRI scans are other noninvasive diagnostic tests that aid in the diagnosis of an aneurysm. Invasive studies, such as digital subtraction an-

Clinical Findings Associated with Abdominal, Thoracic, and Dissecting Aortic Aneurysms

Abdominal Aneurysm

Gnawing pain in hypogastrium and lower back
Full feeling in epigastrium
Pulsatile mass over aorta
Abdominal bruit

Thoracic Aneurysm

Tracheal deviation
Wheezing, cough, dyspnea, stridor
Hemoptysis
Hoarseness
Dysphagia
Pain in chest or back

Dissecting Aneurysm

Ripping or tearing pain
Diaphoresis
Nausea or vomiting
Faintness
Signs and symptoms of ventricular dysfunction
Pulse deficit
Murmur of aortic insufficiency
Neurologic manifestations
Hypertension

giography and arteriography, may provide other necessary diagnostic information. Refer to Chapter 2 for additional information about diagnostic tests.

Treatment

Medical treatment of an aneurysm consists of monitoring the patient for signs of expansion or impending rupture and controlling the patient's blood pressure. High blood pressure not only increases the risk of aneurysm rupture but also accelerates the atherosclerotic degeneration of the vessel. Typically, medical management is reserved for the patient with a small aneurysm or one who is not a surgical candidate. In most situations, surgical removal of the aneurysm or repair of the dissection is the treatment of choice. The risks of surgery include hemorrhage and ischemia to end organs and structures, such as the kidney, bowel, and spinal cord.

A primary objective for the patient with an aneurysm is to maintain optimal hemodynamic stability. Special concerns for the postsurgical patient include adequate volume status to maintain flow through the graft and minimize ischemic damage; adequate distal circulation, since thrombus or embolic debris released at the time of surgery may decrease blood flow; adequate cardiac function, since many of these patients have concomitant coronary artery disease and are at risk for myocardial infarction, congestive failure, and dysrhythmias; and adequate perfusion to maintain renal, gastrointestinal, and spinal cord function, since ischemia is a risk while the aorta is clamped during surgery. Additionally, control of high blood pressure is important to prevent leaking at the anastomotic sites.

Clinical Alert

Sudden onset of pain or a ripping or tearing sensation may indicate rupture of an aneurysm, which is an emergency situation.

Thrombophlebitis

Overview

Thrombophlebitis refers to inflammation of a vein with formation of a clot or thrombus. Predisposing factors for thrombophlebitis include the following triad: venous stasis, trauma to the vein intima, and hypercoagulability of the blood. Increased risk for thrombophlebitis occurs with surgery, bedrest, trauma of the extremities, heart disease, varicose veins, and oral contraceptives. Since most thrombophlebitis occurs in the deep veins of the legs, a major concern is dislodgement of the thrombus, resulting in a pulmonary embolism.

Major Subjective/Objective Data

Common signs and symptoms associated with thrombophlebitis include warmth, redness, edema, and increased size of the extremity; tenderness over the vein with palpation; Homan's sign (although of low sensitivity and specificity); skin changes, such as mottling or cyanosis; and a palpable venous "cord."

In some instances, signs and symptoms of pulmonary embolism may be the first indication of a venous problem. Findings associated with pulmonary embolism include anxiety and restlessness, dyspnea, cough, pleuritic chest pain, hemoptysis, tachycardia, tachypnea, right ventricular strain (RV heave, increased P_2, gallop), rubs, crackles, and wheezes. If the embolus is massive, sudden shock will occur.

Diagnostic Tests

The venous Doppler examination and impedance plethysmography (IPG) help to identify decreased venous flow in the affected extremity, which is suggestive of thrombosis. Other diagnostic tests include radioiodine fibrinogen scanning and nuclide venography. A contrast venogram provides the most definitive information about the location and extent of the thrombus. If pulmonary embolism is suspected, a pulmonary ventilation perfusion scan may be helpful in the diagnosis. Pulmonary angiography is the definitive study for diagnosis of pulmonary embolism. Refer to Chapter 2 for additional information on diagnostic tests.

Treatment

Nonpharmacologic therapy for deep vein thrombophlebitis includes bedrest, application of heat, elevation of the extremity, and use of support stockings and devices. Pharmacologic therapy includes antiinflammatory agents and anticoagulation agents, initially with heparin and later with warfarin. In addition, thrombolytic agents may be used in select cases.

If anticoagulation is contraindicated or if pulmonary embolism occurs despite anticoagulation, surgical interruption of the inferior vena cava may be necessary. Techniques used include insertion of an inferior vena cava umbrella, plication of the inferior vena cava, and clipping the inferior vena cava.

The goals of care focus on patient comfort, elimination and control of predisposing factors for thrombus formation, and prevention and treatment of pulmonary embolism. Patient care responsibilities include careful assessment and evaluation of the patient's response to therapy, including monitoring for both overt and covert signs of bleeding secondary to anticoagulation. Additionally, the patient needs to be educated on the reduction of predisposing factors for thromboembolism and precautions to be taken with anticoagulation.

Clinical Alert

Monitor for acute onset of chest pain, dyspnea, tachypnea, and hemodynamic instability, which may be indicators of pulmonary embolism.

Selected bibliography

Braunwald E, editor: *Heart disease: a textbook of cardiovascular medicine,* Philadelphia, 1992, Saunders.

Dolan J: Critical care nursing, Philadelphia, 1991, FA Davis.

Frolich E: Current issues in hypertension: old questions with new answers and new questions, *Medical Clinics of North America* 76(5):1043-1056, 1992.

Genest J and others: Lipoprotein cholesterol, apolipoprotein A-I and B and lipoprotein (a) abnormalities in men with premature coronary artery disease, *Journal of the American College of Cardiology* 19(4):792-802, 1992.

Guzzetta C, Dossey B: *Cardiovascular nursing—holistic practice* St Louis, 1992, Mosby.

Hurst JW, editor: *The heart, arteries and veins,* New York, 1990, McGraw-Hill.

Israel D, Gorlin R: Fish oils in the prevention of atherosclerosis, *Journal of American College of Cardiology* 19(1):174-185, 1992.

Kinney M and others: *Comprehensive cardiac care,* ed 7, St Louis, 1991, Mosby.

Kinney M, Packa D, Dunbar S: *AACN's clinical reference for critical care nursing,* ed 3, New York, 1993, McGraw-Hill.

Matrisciono L: Unstable angina: an overview, *Critical Care Nurse* 12(8):30-40, 1992.

Stewart S: Acute MI: A review of pathophysiology, treatment, and complications, *Journal of Cardiovascular Nursing* 6(4):1-25, 1992.

Swearingen P, Keen J, editors: *Manual of critical care,* St Louis, 1991, Mosby.

The fifth report of the joint National Committee on detection, evaluation, and treatment of high blood pressure, Bethesda, Maryland, January 1993, National Institues of Health.

Cardiovascular Assessment

2

Subjective Data

A careful analysis of symptoms can reveal information about the patient's baseline status and progression of the disease. Investigating the anatomic location, quality, quantity and time sequence of the symptom(s), precipitating and alleviating factors, and any concomitant symptoms can assist the health care provider in analysis of the problem and development of a plan of care (Table 2-1).

Objective Data

Objective data collection requires a physical assessment of the body's systems to identify signs associated with cardiovascular disorders. Findings can also validate and amplify the subjective data collected from the patient.

General Appearance

Evaluate the degree of distress or discomfort and outward manifestations, such as facial expression, posture, and reactions to the environment.

Head/Neck

Inspection

Note color of skin and mucous membranes. Inspect eyes for xanthelasma, arcus corneae, and funduscopic changes. Inspect neck veins for jugular venous distention (JVD). See p. 132.

- To differentiate carotid pulse from jugular vein pulsation, check the carotid pulse during respiration or while changing position. Carotid pulsations are not affected by these maneu-

Table 2-1 Common presenting complaints

Chest pain	Can be cardiac or noncardiac in origin (see Table 2-2).
Dyspnea	Subjective sensation of being unable to breathe.
Orthopnea	Ability to breathe only in an upright position.
Paroxysmal nocturnal dyspnea	Sudden inability to breathe occurring during sleep.
Cough	A dry, irritating, spasmodic cough is usually associated with cardiovascular disorders. Frothy, pink-tinged sputum occurs in pulmonary edema.
Palpitations	Patient awareness of heart rhythm abnormalities; referred to as "pounding," "fluttering," "racing," or "skipped beats."
Dizziness/syncope	Lightheadedness, temporary loss of consciousness; may be related to heart block, pacemaker malfunction, aortic stenosis, dysrhythmias, or hypovolemia.
Edema	Fluid accumulation in the interstitial spaces; may be related to congestive heart failure, venous insufficiency, or noncardiac disorders.
Fatigue	Generalized feeling of tiredness associated with a variety of disorders; may be related to decreased cardiac output, drugs, electrolyte imbalance.
Nocturia	Urination at night, common in congestive heart failure secondary to increased redistribution of fluids associated with the supine position.
Claudication	Pain related to arterial insufficiency that can occur in the arch of the foot, calf, thigh, or buttocks. May be a cramp, ache, or numb feeling.

Table 2-2 Differentiating chest pain

Pain	Associated Symptoms	Relieving Factors
Angina		
Retrosternal, diffuse discomfort. May radiate to jaw, neck, arms, back, or upper abdomen. Onset is gradual or sudden. Usually lasts < 15 minutes. Physical or emotional factors and exposure to hot or cold temperatures can precipitate attack. Angina can occur at rest or with activity.	Dyspnea Indigestion Sweating Dizziness Syncope Anxiety	Removal of cause Rest Nitroglycerin
Myocardial Infarction		
Onset is sudden; pain lasts > 30 minutes. May have no precipitating factors.	Same as angina Pulmonary congestion and extra heart sounds may also be present	May or may not be relieved by narcotics

Continued.

Table 2-2   Differentiating chest pain—cont'd

Pain	Associated Symptoms	Relieving Factors
Dissecting Aortic Aneurysm		
Anterior chest pain that can radiate to back and abdomen. Pain shifts as the dissection progresses. Pain is excruciating and may have a "tearing" sensation. Onset is sudden and pain can last for hours. High blood pressure is a precipitating factor.	Apprehension Dyspnea Diaphoresis BP differs between arms Pulses may be absent Murmur of aortic insufficiency may be present	Pharmacologic agents to control blood pressure Narcotics may relieve pain
Pericarditis		
Pain is precordial or substernal. May radiate to shoulders and neck. Onset is sudden. May be precipitated by myocardial infarction, trauma, infection, or uremia.	Dyspnea Tachypnea Pericardial friction rub Deep breathing, coughing, and supine position increases pain	Leaning forward Nonsteroidal antiinflammatory agents
Pulmonary Embolus		
Pleuritic chest pain is associated with pulmonary infarction with or without dys-	Dyspnea Tachypnea	Narcotics

pnea. Dyspnea and tachypnea may be the only signs of pulmonary embolus, or signs of cardiac failure may develop. Onset is sudden. Deep vein thrombosis may be a precipitating factor.	Apprehension Hemoptysis Crackles Hypotension Pleural rub Tachycardia Syncope Cardiac arrest Right-sided heart failure	
Musculoskeletal Disorders		
Localized pain. Onset is sudden or gradual. May be intermittent or continuous. Strain is a precipitating factor.	Movement increases pain, soreness	Rest Heat Analgesics
Gastrointestinal Disorders		
Pain in epigastric area. May radiate to back, upper abdomen, or shoulder. Onset may be sudden or gradual. Pain may be intermittent or continuous. Precipitated by alcohol, foods, medications, recumbent position.	Belching Dysphagia Nausea Vomiting	Antacids Belching Sitting upright H_2 antagonists

vers. Jugular pulsations descend with inspiration and increase in a recumbent position.
- Carotid pulses are palpable; venous pulses are not.
- Normal JVD is 3 cm (1½ inches) or less.

Palpation

Palpate the carotid arteries to determine quality, rate, and equality of pulses and thrills.
- Palpate pulses (*except* carotid pulse) bilaterally and simultaneously.
- Carotid pulse is the best indicator of cardiac function.

Auscultation

- Auscultate the carotid arteries with the bell of the stethoscope while the patient holds his or her breath.
- The optimum location for listening to venous hum is directly over the supraclavicular space; with the patient in a sitting position. Venous hum is loudest in diastole and can disappear when pressure is applied to the jugular vein. A venous hum is not indicative of disease but must be differentiated from cardiac murmurs and bruits.

Thorax

Inspection

Assess the shape, size, wall movement, rate of respiration, breathing pattern, and use of accessory muscles.

Auscultation

Auscultate the lung fields: anterior, posterior, and lateral. Note crackles, wheezes, and decreased or absent breath sounds.

Precordium

Inspection

Inspect for heaves or lifts, pulsations, and retractions.
- Examine all areas of the precordium.
- Apical impulse is the only pulsation normally visible.

Palpation

Palpate for heaves or lifts, thrills, and apical impulse.
- Use fingertips to palpate pulsations.
- Apical impulse is located at the fifth left intercostal space midclavicular line, an area <2 cm in diameter.

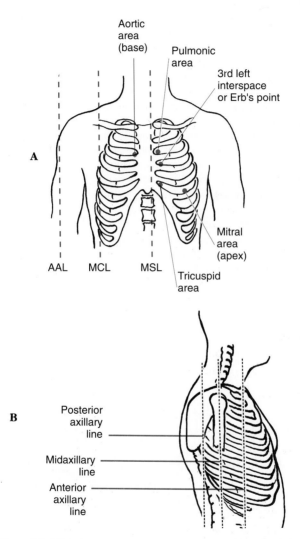

Figure 2-1 A,B

Cardiac auscultatory areas and anatomic landmarks. *AAL*, Anterior axillary line; *MCL*, midclavicular line; *MSL*, midsternal line.

Auscultation

Auscultate apical pulse and note rate and rhythm; assess heart sounds and note any extra cardiac sounds (Figures 2-1 and 2-2, Table 2-3). Evaluate for murmurs (Tables 2-4, 2-5, and 1-20).

- Systematically auscultate each area of the precordium and concentrate on one component of the cardiac cycle at a time, then listen for the presence of extra sounds and murmurs.
- Count irregular heart rhythm for 1 full minute. Determine existence of apical-radial deficit.
- The bell accentuates lower frequency sounds—S_3, S_4.
- The diaphragm accentuates high-frequency sounds—S_1, S_2.
- Describe murmurs in regard to location, distance from midsternal, midclavicular, or axillary lines (see Figure 2-1).
- Document murmur according to

  Timing: systole, diastole

  Intensity: grade of murmur (see Table 2-5)

  Quality: harsh, blowing, or rumbling

  Location: aortic, pulmonic, tricuspid, or mitral areas

  Radiation: axilla, neck, or sternal border

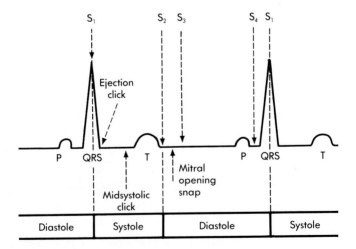

Figure 2-2

Heart sounds in relation to ECG.

Table 2-3 Differentiating heart sounds

Heart Sound	Best Area to Auscultate	Description	Mechanism	Timing
S_1	Apex	Normally $S_1 > S_2$; does not vary with respirations	Mitral and tricuspid valve closure	Systole
S_2	Base	Normally $S_2 > S_1$ at aortic area	Aortic and pulmonic valve closure	Diastole
S_3	Apex, LSB	Abnormal in adults; referred to as ventricular gallop	Diastolic overload of ventricles; decreased ventricular compliance	Early diastole; after S_2
S_4	Apex, LSB	Usually abnormal; referred to as atrial gallop; increases with inspiration	Systolic overload of ventricles; decreased ventricular compliance	Late diastole; before S_1
Summation gallop		Atrial and ventricular gallops occur simultaneously		Mid diastole
Split S_1	4ICS, LSB	Normal in most cases	Mitral valve closes slightly before tricuspid valve because of higher pressure gradient on left side of heart	Systole

Continued.

Table 2-3   Differentiating heart sounds—cont'd

Heart Sound	Best Area to Auscultate	Description	Mechanism	Timing
Split S$_2$	Pulmonic area; 2ICS, LSB	Normal if corresponds to respiratory cycle; possibly abnormal if occurs during expiration	Pulmonic valve closes later than aortic valve during inspiration because of increased venous return	End of systole
Aortic ejection sound	2ICS, RSB; Apex	Abnormal; aortic ejection sound does not change with respiration	Ejection of blood from left ventricle through a diseased aortic valve	Early systole
Pulmonic ejection sound	2ICS, LSB	Pulmonic ejection sound increases in intensity with expiration and decreases with inspiration	Ejection of blood from right ventricle through a diseased pulmonary valve	Early systole

Midsystolic click	Apex	Associated with mitral valve prolapse; decreases in intensity or absent at base	Sudden tension on chordae and prolapsing leaflets	Midsystole to late systole
Opening snap (OS)	Lower LSB, 4ICS	Abnormal; can be differentiated from S_3 because it occurs earlier in the cardiac cycle, is higher pitched, and radiates more widely. Differentiated from split S_2 by area where it is best heard. OS not affected by respiration	Opening of stenotic mitral valve	Early diastole
Pericardial friction rub	Loudest along LSB	Abnormal; usually a result of pericarditis	Rubbing of inflamed surfaces of pericardial sac	Systole and diastole

ICS, intercostal space. LSB, left sternal border. RSB, right sternal border.

Table 2-4 **Murmurs and related valvular disorders**

Timing	Valvular Disorder	Auscultatory Location	Quality
Holosystolic; occurs throughout S_1 and S_2	Mitral insufficiency	Apex; often radiates to left axilla or back	High-pitched; blowing; plateau
	Tricuspid insufficiency	LLSB	High-pitched; blowing; intensity increases during inspiration
Systole (systolic ejection murmur); occurs between S_1 and S_2	Aortic stenosis	2 RICS; may radiate to apex and neck	Harsh; crescendo-decrescendo
	Pulmonic stenosis	2 LICS; may radiate to left side of neck	Harsh; crescendo-decrescendo
Early diastole; onset is immediately after S_2	Aortic insufficiency	3 LICS and LSB; best heard when patient sitting up leaning forward; may radiate to R or L of sternum	High-pitched; blowing; decrescendo
Mid diastole to late diastole; onset is more mid-diastole or later	Pulmonic insufficiency	2 LICS; 3 LICS	Blowing; decrescendo
	Mitral stenosis	PMI	Rumbling; crescendo-decrescendo
	Tricuspid stenosis	LLSB	Rumbling; increases in intensity with inspiration; crescendo-decrescendo

LLSB, lower left sternal border. RICS, right intercostal space. LICS, left intercostal space. L, left. R, right. PMI, point of maximal impulse.

Table 2-5   **Murmur intensity**

Grade	Description
I/VI	Faint, heard after a period of concentration
II/VI	Soft, faint, heard immediately on auscultation
III/VI	Moderate intensity, heard well
IV/VI	Loud murmur with thrill
V/VI	Loud, requiring a stethoscope
VI/VI	Very loud, can be heard with stethoscope off chest

- A systolic ejection murmur at the second left intercostal space is normal in high flow states.
- Diastolic and continuous murmurs are always pathologic.
- Sudden appearance of holosystolic murmur along the left sternal border or apex in a patient with an MI may indicate rupture of the ventricular septum or a papillary muscle.
- Acute decompensation in patients with valve replacements may develop without any auscultatory abnormalities.

Abdomen

Inspection

Inspect for size, shape, distention, pulsations, and ascites.
- Measure abdominal girth at the umbilicus during expiration. Mark the area to be measured to ensure consistency and accuracy of measurement.

Auscultation

Auscultate aorta and renal, iliac, and femoral arteries; inferior vena cava; liver and spleen.
- Auscultate abdomen before beginning palpation.

Palpation

Palpate the liver, aorta, and femoral pulses.
- If right-sided heart failure is suspected but resting venous pressures are normal, the hepatojugular reflex test (HJR) is indicated. Press the upper right quadrant of the abdomen for 30 to 60 seconds while observing the neck veins. An increase

- > 3 cm indicates a positive HJR. To ensure accuracy, the patient should breathe normally during the test and the head of the bed must be positioned at a 45° angle.
- Aorta is normally 2.5 to 4.0 cm wide.

Extremities

Inspection

Inspect the skin for color, pigmentation, texture, lesions, edema, hair distribution, and varicosities; the nailbeds for color and clubbing; and the dorsal hand veins for an estimate of venous pressure. See p. 132.

Palpation

Palpate skin, noting temperature, moisture, turgor; calf tenderness (determine presence or absence of Homan's sign); edema (Table 2-6); and capillary refill. Palpate pulses (radial, brachial, femoral, popliteal, dorsalis pedis, posterior tibialis). Note rate, rhythm, and amplitude (3+ bounding, 2+ normal, 1+ weak, 0 absent).

- Capillary refill should be < 3 seconds.
- Use thumb to assess depth of pitting edema.
- Simultaneously palpate pulses bilaterally.
- Mark location of pulses with a pen or marker when pulses are difficult to find.
- If unable to palpate pulses, use the doppler.
- Dorsalis pedis pulse is absent or nonpalpable in about 10% of the population.
- Closely monitor pulses distal to arterial catheters; if decreased or absent, notify physician.

Auscultation

Check blood pressure in both of the patient's arms while patient is supine and standing. Calculate mean arterial pressure and the pulse

Table 2-6   **Assessing pitting edema**

Degree of Edema	Grade	Depth of Depression
Mild	1+	<¼ inch
Moderate	2+	¼-½ inch
Severe	3+	½-1 inch

pressure (see Appendix B). Determine the presence or absence of pulsus paradoxus (see p. 138).

- Use a blood pressure cuff that is 20% wider than the diameter of the limb. A cuff that is too small will result in a falsely high pressure reading; a cuff that is too large will result in a falsely low reading.
- Determine palpatory systolic pressure before auscultating BP (see procedure on p. 138).

Findings Associated with Cardiovascular Problems

Adventitious heart sounds

Adventitious heart sounds are abnormal. An S_3 is a hallmark for congestive heart failure (see Table 2-3).

Arcus corneae

This finding is characterized by a thin gray or white ring located in the corneal region. It is normal in the elderly and in blacks. If observed in young whites, it may be related to premature atherosclerosis.

Arterial/venous insufficiency

See Table 2-7 for ways to differentiate between arterial and venous insufficiency.

Arteriovenous nicking

Arteriovenous nicking is a finding associated with arteriosclerosis, high blood pressure and diabetes mellitus. When the fundus of the eye is examined, the vein appears to stop on either side of the arteriole (normally, arteriolar walls are invisible and veins are visible up to either side of the arteriole).

Ascites

Ascites, an abnormal accumulation of fluid within the peritoneal cavity, may be associated with heart failure and constrictive pericarditis.

Blood pressure

Increased blood pressure may be related to increased demand for cardiac output, which may in turn be caused by stress, pain, hypoxia, drugs, or a disease process.

Decreased blood pressure may be related to bedrest, drugs, dysrhythmias, shock, or myocardial infarction.

✗ Table 2-7   **Differentiating arterial/venous insufficiency**

	Arterial	Venous
Pain	Upon walking	While standing
Pain relief	Resting, standing, or dependent positioning of lower extremity	Elevation of extremity
Swelling	None	Present
Pulses	Decreased, absent	May be difficult to palpate with edematous foot
Integument changes	Hair loss, skin shiny, nail thickening	Brownish pigment
	Cool to touch	Normal temperature
	Pallor when extremity elevated, dependent rubor (reactive hyperemia)	May be cyanotic when extremity in dependent position
	Ulcers located on toes or site of trauma	Ulcers located on side of ankle or pretibial area
	Gangrene possible	

Unequal blood pressure—differences in blood pressure between the arms or the legs may indicate coarctation of the aorta, aortic dissection, or subclavian steal syndrome. A difference in blood pressure of 10 mm Hg between the arms is normal. Blood pressure in the legs is normally 10 mm Hg higher than that in the arms.

Orthostatic blood pressure is a drop of 10 to 15 mm Hg in systolic blood pressure and 10 mm Hg in diastolic blood pressure upon standing. It is associated with an increase in heart rate of 10 to 20 beats per minute. Orthostatic blood pressure may be related to hypovolemia, drugs, or prolonged bedrest.

Bruits

An abnormal sound or murmur associated with atherosclerosis is classified as a bruit. Bruits do not necessarily signify disease if auscultated over the aorta. However, if associated with absent pulses in the legs, they may indicate a dissecting aneurysm. Bruits may be a sign of an obstructive lesion in the renal arteries if auscultated over the kidney area.

Cheyne-Stokes respirations

A breathing pattern characterized by hyperpnea and apnea, Cheyne-Stokes respirations are a late sign of congestive heart failure.

Clubbing

Clubbing is the loss of the 20° angle at the base of the nail; it is associated with chronic oxygen deficiency.

Crackles

Crackles are abnormal breath sounds that indicate fluid in the airways. These wet or dry crackling sounds not relieved by coughing may be associated with congestive heart failure.

Cyanosis

Central cyanosis is characterized by a bluish color of the tongue and mucous membranes inside of the cheeks. It results from low arterial oxygen saturation. Peripheral cyanosis is characterized by bluish lips and is associated with exposure to cold or low cardiac output related to heart failure. Arterial oxygen saturation is normal.

Dorsal hand veins

Dorsal hand veins provide a rough estimate of venous pressure. If it takes > 3 to 5 seconds for veins to fill when the arm is dependent, suspect hypovolemia. Distention of veins when the arm is elevated above the sternal angle indicates elevated venous pressure. (See p. 132.)

Edema

Edema is the visible excess of interstitial fluid. Unilateral edema is associated with local factors, such as varicose veins and thrombophlebitis. Bilateral edema can be associated with congestive heart failure.

Heave

A heave is a sustained apical impulse. If located at the fifth LICS, MCL, it is associated with left ventricular hypertrophy. A sustained apical impulse at the third to fourth LICS is associated with right ventricular hypertrophy. When generalized over the entire precordium, it is associated with mitral regurgitation.

Hepatojugular reflux

Hepatojugular reflux is a test to observe distention of the jugular vein induced by manual pressure over the liver. The test result is abnormal if venous pressure increases > 3 cm and suggests insufficiency of the right side of the heart.

Hepatomegaly

Hepatomegaly, or enlargement of the liver, may be associated with heart failure or constrictive pericarditis.

Homan's sign

Homan's sign is defined as calf pain with dorsiflexion of the foot and is suggestive of thrombophlebitis.

Hums

Generally an innocent sign, hums are continuous murmurs that disappear when pressure is applied over the vein. Hums may be related to tumor or veno-obstructive processes if auscultated over the liver and spleen.

Hyperkinetic pulse

Hyperkinetic pulse is a bounding pulse usually produced by an increased stroke volume.

Hypokinetic pulse

Hypokinetic pulse is a weak pulse usually produced by a low cardiac output.

Jaundice

Defined as yellowing of sclerae or skin, jaundice may be related to hemolysis of red blood cells associated with patients who have prosthetic valves.

Jugular venous distention

JVD > 3 cm is suggestive of fluid volume excess. CVP > 12 cm H_2O or 8 mm Hg may be associated with heart failure or pericardial disease. CVP < 5 cm H_2O or 2 mm Hg may be associated with hypovolemia.

Kussmaul's sign

A paradoxic rise in level of jugular vein distention during inspiration, Kussmaul's sign, may be related to constrictive pericarditis.

Lesions

Osler's nodes are tender, raised nodules that are reddish purple with white centers. They are located on the distal pads of fingers, toes, palms of hands, or soles of feet. They are associated with bacterial endocarditis.

Janeway lesions are raised, erythematous, macular skin lesions on palms of hands or soles of feet that are associated with bacterial endocarditis.

Xanthoma is a papule, nodule, or plaque in the skin made up of lipid deposits and associated with increased cholesterol levels.

Ecchymosis is a bruise in the skin associated with thrombocytopenia, trauma, and steroid therapy.

Splinter hemorrhage is a subungual hemorrhage that resembles a splinter of wood. It is found in a small percentage of patients with bacterial endocarditis.

Petechiae are capillary hemorrhages. Usually < 2 mm in size, they are associated with blood dyscrasias.

Varicose veins are prominent dilatations and irregularities of leg veins associated with heart failure, thrombophlebitis, and incompetent vein valves.

Mean arterial pressure

Mean arterial pressure is an index of perfusion pressure. A pressure > 105 mm Hg may be related to high blood pressure or vasoconstriction; a pressure < 70 mm Hg may be related to vasodilation or hypotension. A decreased MAP may cause coronary artery graft collapse and decreased renal function.

Moisture

Diaphoresis is excess sweating associated with decreased cardiac output and sympathetic nervous system response.

Murmurs

Diastolic and continuous murmurs are always pathologic. Prosthetic valves produce systolic (aortic valve prosthesis) and diastolic (mitral valve prosthesis) murmurs. A holosystolic murmur along the LSB is associated with a ventricular septal defect (VSD) (see Table 2-4).

Pallor

Pallor is a loss of rosy pink color that may be associated with hypoxia, vasoconstriction, or anemia.

Pulsations

Pulsations may be normal in the epigastric area. Exaggerated pulsations can be indicative of abdominal aortic aneurysm or right ventricular hypertrophy.

Displacement downward and to the left of the apex is associated with left ventricular dilatation. When present at the third to fourth ICS LSB, pulsations are associated with right ventricular enlargement. When present at the second LICS, they are associated with a dilated pulmonary artery. When present at the upper right sternal edge, they are associated with dilatation or aneurysm of the aortic root. When present at the third to fourth LICS MCL, they are associated with bulging of the ischemic or aneurysmal anterior surface of the left ventricle.

Pulse pressure

Pulse pressure is the difference between systolic and diastolic blood pressure. It reflects stroke volume.

Pulse pressure > 50 mm Hg may be related to arteriosclerosis, fluid overload, increased stroke volume, or aortic insufficiency.

Pulse pressure < 30 mm Hg may be related to decreased stroke volume, coarctation of the aorta, or drugs.

Pulses

Bradycardia is a heart rate of < 60 beats per minute. It may be related to drugs, vagal stimuli, or MI. Bradycardia may adversely affect cardiac output.

Tachycardia is a heart rate of > 100 beats per minute. It may be related to anemia, anxiety, fever, drugs, decreased stroke volume, or congestive heart failure. Tachycardia can adversely affect cardiac output.

Pulse deficit is the difference between the radial and apical pulse rate. It may be related to atrial fibrillation or decreased blood flow through the radial artery.

Irregular rhythm is related to dysrhythmias, such as atrial fibrillation or flutter, premature beats, and heart block.

Absent/unequal pulse is related to arterial insufficiency, atherosclerosis, emboli, or dissecting aortic aneurysm. See Table 3-1 for a visualization of pulse variations and associated disorders.

Pulsus paradoxus

Pulsus paradoxus is a fall in systolic blood pressure > 10 mm Hg during inspiration; it is associated with constrictive pericarditis, acute cardiac tamponade, and severe obstructive lung disease.

Retraction

An inward movement of the apical impulse during systole, retraction may be associated with constrictive pericarditis.

Rubor

Rubor is a red color usually accompanied by systemic vasodilation.

Temperature

Temperature increases with dehydration or infection. It may be elevated for the first few days following MI. Fever increases demand on the heart.

Temperature decreases with decreased blood flow to an area, as in the case of shock or heart failure. Hypothermia is induced during cardiac surgery.

Thrills

These palpable sensations provide no diagnostic information other than the presence of a murmur.

Xanthelasma

Xanthelasma is characterized by lipid deposits on the eyelids and is associated with atherosclerosis.

Fluid Volume Assessment

Cardiac dysfunction can cause excess extracellular fluid volume, which in turn can further decrease myocardial function. Diuretic agents are prescribed to help eliminate excess fluid volume. However, aggressive therapy may result in a volume deficit. Thus fluid

Table 2-8   **Signs and symptoms associated with volume disturbances**

	Hypovolemia	Hypervolemia
Weight	Acute loss	Acute gain
Pulse	Tachycardia	Bounding pulse
Blood pressure	Postural hypotension	Hypertension
	Decreased pulse pressure	
Mucous membranes	Dry	Moist
Turgor	Decreased skin elasticity	Pitting edema
	Furrowed tongue	
Peripheral veins	Neck veins flat when supine	JVP elevated
	Slow filling of hand veins	
Hemodynamics	CVP < 2 cm H_2O	CVP > 12 cm H_2O
	Decreased PAWP	Increased PAWP
Other	Thirst	Cough
	Urine output < 30 ml/hr	Dyspnea
		Crackles
		S_3
		Pulmonary edema
Laboratory data	Increased hemoglobin	Decreased hemoglobin
	Increased hematocrit	Decreased hematocrit
	Increased serum osmolality	Decreased serum osmolality
	Increased specific gravity	Decreased specific gravity
	Increased BUN:creatinine ratio	

JVP, jugular venous pressure. CVP, central venous pressure. PAWP, pulmonary artery wedge pressure.

volume assessment is important in cardiac patients so that imbalances can be detected early and treatment initiated. Table 2-8 describes signs and symptoms associated with volume disturbances.

- 1 kg equals 1 liter of fluid; a gain of 0.25 to 0.5 kg/day reflects excess fluid.
- 10 to 15 lb of fluid can accumulate before edema is apparent.
- Daily weights should be done at the same time of the day, with the same amount of clothing and on the same scale.
- Check mucous membranes at the area where the cheek and gum meet; this area is not affected by mouth breathing.
- The best area to assess skin turgor is the sternum, forehead, or inner aspects of the thigh.
- Maintain accurate intake and output records; normally, intake should approximate output.
- Fever increases fluid loss.
- Urine output should be 1 ml/kg/hour; less output is common during stress.
- Record the intake of ice chips (fluid volume is half of the amount of ice chips).
- A rough estimate of serum osmolality can be calculated using the following formula: 2(Na) + Glucose/18 + BUN/3. Normal is 280 to 295 mOsm/kg; > 295 is indicative of dehydration; < 280 is indicative of overhydration.

Psychosocial Assessment

The chronic nature of cardiovascular disease coupled with the constant potential for a life-threatening event can cause psychologic and social stress in the individual. Strained relationships, depleted finances, lack of understanding of the disease and therapeutic regimen, and inability to cope are but a few problems that can occur. In addition, some of these psychosocial factors can adversely affect cardiovascular function (i.e., fear, anxiety, and the inability to cope with the disease may increase the sympathetic response and increase the demand on the heart).

Cognitive: Orientation, Memory, Learning Needs, Comprehension

Is the patient alert, drowsy, confused, oriented? Can the patient remember events? Does the patient understand what is going on? Does the patient understand the disease and treatment?

Response to Health and Illness: Perception, Support, Coping Style, Culture

What is the patient's understanding of the illness? What does it mean to the patient? Are there effective support systems? What is the patient's relationship with the family? How does this illness affect the family? Does the patient have financial concerns? How is the patient coping? Are there signs of anxiety, depression, hostility, acceptance, powerlessness, loneliness, fear? Does the patient adhere to rituals, practices, or beliefs that influence health behavior?

Sensory-Perceptual Integration: Sleep, Overload, Deprivation

Is the patient getting adequate sleep and rest? What are the environmental factors affecting the patient? Are environmental stimuli meaningful? Is the patient receiving any medications that may cause sensory impairment?

Other Bedside Assessment Parameters

Assessment of the therapies and data obtained by special monitoring devices is important to the development of a comprehensive and accurate data base.

Intravenous Infusions

Assess and document:
1. Type of solution
2. Rate of infusion
3. Site location and appearance
4. Infusion device alarm function

Hemodynamic Monitoring

Assess and document:
1. Site location and appearance
2. Circulation to extremity (when indicated)
3. Proper placement of transducer
4. Calibration of equipment
5. Waveform and pressures
6. Alarm function

See Chapter 3 for specifics on hemodynamic monitoring.

Clinical Alert

- Place transducer at phlebostatic axis.
- Read RA, PA, and LA pressures at end expiration.
- Observe for PA catheter displacement, i.e., permanent "wedge" tracing; right ventricular tracing; or dysrhythmias, such as premature ventricular beats or ventricular tachycardia.
- Do not inflate balloon of PA catheter with fluid.
- Allow balloon to deflate passively.
- Do not keep balloon inflated for more than 15 seconds.
- Evaluate trends of pressure readings, not just a single reading.

Cardiac Monitoring

Assess and document:
1. Lead placement
2. Rate, rhythm
3. Rate alarm function

Clinical Alert

- Ground all electrical equipment.
- Ensure good skin contact of electrode.
- Avoid placement of electrodes near potential defibrillator pad placement.

Oxygen Therapy

Assess and document:
1. Method of administration
2. Flow rate; FIo_2
3. Ventilator settings
4. Ventilator alarms

Clinical Alert

- Ensure humidified O_2.
- Avoid flow rates > 2L (nasal cannula or prongs) if patient has COPD.
- Tell patient and visitors not to smoke while oxygen is in use.
- Keep manual resuscitator available for emergency use.

Wounds

Assess and document:
1. Location
2. Appearance

3. Amount and quality of drainage
4. Presence or absence of dressing

Drainage Devices

Assess and document:
1. Type (nasogastric tube, chest tube, Penrose drain, urinary catheter, etc.)
2. Tube location and patency
3. Skin condition
4. Amount and description of drainage
5. Type and amount of suction (if indicated)

Clinical Alert

· Notify physician immediately if > 100 ml per hour or sudden cessation of chest tube drainage occurs in the immediate postoperative cardiac patient.
· Urine output of < 0.5 to 1.0 ml/kg/hour may reflect decreased cardiac output (see Appendix C).

Electrical Safety

Assess high risk situations:
1. Equipment—exposed or frayed wires, broken plugs, two-prong plugs, wet items on top of monitors or equipment
2. Bed—electric, wet linens
3. Floor—wet with blood or other fluids
4. Temporary pacemaker—exposed wires
5. Intravascular lines—direct access to heart

Clinical Alert

· Correct or eliminate risk factor(s) when possible.
· Touch bed rails before touching patients with pacemakers or intravascular lines.
· Ground all metal beds.
· Use equipment with a visible, approved inspection tag.
· Wear rubber gloves when handling generator or leads of temporary pacemakers.
· Cap exposed pacemaker wires.

Laboratory Tests

Laboratory tests can provide important information in the assessment, diagnosis, and management of cardiovascular disease. Selected tests and their cardiovascular implications are presented in the following pages.

Blood Chemistry

Blood chemistry tests are used to evaluate the effects of cardiac disease and also to identify chemical imbalances that may compromise cardiovascular function (Table 2-9).

Coagulation Studies

Coagulation studies aid in the diagnosis of hemostasis problems. They are also valuable for monitoring the effects of anticoagulation and thrombolytic therapy (Table 2-10).

Clinical Alert

Monitor for covert as well as overt bleeding if results from coagulation studies fall outside the normal ranges.

Enzymes

Enzymes are used to diagnose a variety of disorders, including myocardial infarction. Information about enzymes that have specific cardiovascular significance can be found in Tables 2-11 and 2-12.

Clinical Alert

Other causes of enzyme elevations include intramuscular injections, thrombolytic therapy, and cardiac trauma (cardioversion or defibrillation, cardiac surgery).

Hematology

Select hematological studies are useful in the assessment of cardiac workload and identification of myocardial damage (Table 2-13).

Blood Gases

Blood gases reflect not only acid-base status but also oxygen saturation of the blood. Acid-base imbalance, whether acidosis or alkalosis, adversely affects myocardial contractility. Pao_2, arterial O_2 saturation, hemoglobin, and cardiac output determine oxygen delivery to the tissues. Venous O_2 saturation reflects oxygen utilization by the tissues. Normal arterial and venous blood gases can be found in Table 2-14. Acid-base imbalances can be found in Table 2-15.

Text continued on p. 93.

Table 2-9 Blood chemistry and associated cardiovascular implications

Test	Normal Value	Cardiovascular Implications
Sodium (Na)	135-148 mEq/L	Low—dilutional with congestive failure; reflects relative excess of water rather than low total body sodium; depletional with some diuretics
Potassium (K)	3.5-5.0 mEq/L	Low—enhances effect of digitalis (increased risk of toxicity); associated with alkalosis (as pH increases 0.1, potassium decreases 0.6 mEq/L); ECG changes: flattened T wave, depressed ST, presence of U wave, prolonged PR and QT; premature ventricular complexes, atrial tachycardia, junctional tachycardia, ventricular tachycardia, and ventricular fibrillation High—associated with acidosis; (as pH decreases 0.1 potassium increases 0.6 mEq/L); ECG changes: absent P waves, prolonged PR, peaked T wave, wide QRS, sinus bradycardia or arrest, first-degree AV block, junctional rhythm, idioventricular rhythm, ventricular tachycardia, ventricular fibrillation or arrest
Chloride (Cl)	98-106 mEq/L	Low—dilutional with congestive failure; depletional with diuretic administration; may cause metabolic alkalosis
Magnesium (Mg)	1.3-2.1 mEq/L	Low—may cause unexplained hypokalemia and hypocalcemia; ECG changes: prolonged PR and QT; broad, flat T waves; premature ventricular complexes; ventricular tachycardia; and ventricular fibrillation High—ECG changes: prolonged PR and QT, widened QRS, bradycardia

Calcium (Ca)	8.5-10.5 mg/dl 4.5-5.5 mEq/L	Low—ECG change: QT prolonged High—increased chance for digitalis toxicity; ECG changes: QT shortened, PR prolonged, QRS widened, bradycardia
Glucose; fasting blood sugar (FBS)	60-100 mg/dl	High—may be due to stress response of myocardial infarction or following cardiac surgery
Blood urea nitrogen (BUN)	7-18 mg/dl	High—impaired renal function secondary to low cardiac output, cardiogenic shock, hypovolemia
Creatinine	0.6-1.2 mg/dl (women) 0.7-1.3 mg/dl (men)	High—impaired renal function
Cholesterol	120-200 mg/dl	High—associated with increased risk of atherosclerosis

Continued.

Table 2-9 Blood chemistry and associated cardiovascular implications—cont'd

Test	Normal Value	Cardiovascular Implications
High-density lipoprotein (HDL)	30-80 mg/dl (women) 30-70 mg/dl (men)	Low—associated with increased risk of atherosclerosis High—seen as "protective" against atherosclerosis
Low-density lipoprotein (LDL)	62-185 mg/dl; ideally < 130 mg/dl	High—associated with increased risk of atherosclerosis
Triglycerides	40-150 mg/dl (age related)	High—with high cholesterol, associated with increased risk for atherosclerosis
Carbon dioxide content (total CO_2)	23-30 mEq/L	Reflects bicarbonate level Low—metabolic acidosis High—metabolic alkalosis

mEq/L, milliequivalents per liter. mg, milligram. dl, deciliter.

Table 2-10 Coagulation studies and associated cardiovascular implications

Test	Normal Value	Cardiovascular Implications
Bleeding time	3-10 min	May be prolonged by aspirin or alcohol ingestion; value > 10 may indicate impaired primary hemostasis
Platelets	150,000-350,000/mm^3	Generally, platelet counts > 50,000/mm^3 are not associated with spontaneous bleeding
Prothrombin time (PT)	10-14 sec; 100%	Used to monitor anticoagulation with warfarin (coumadin); goal is a PT of 1.2-2.0 times normal or INR 2.0-3.0.
Partial thromboplastin time (PTT); activated partial thromboplastin time (APTT)	30-45 sec 16-25 sec	Used to monitor anticoagulation with heparin: goal of anticoagulation is PTT or APTT 1.5-2.5 times normal
Fibrinogen	200-400 mg/dl	Low—increased fibrinolysis High—may be associated with increased risk of myocardial infarction
Fibrin split products (FSP); fibrin degradation products (FDP)	< 3 µg/ml	Increased with extensive clot formation and activation of fibrinolytic system
Plasminogen	21 mg/dl	Low—increased fibrinolysis

mm^3, millimeters cubed. sec, seconds. min, minutes. mg/dl, milligrams per deciliter. µg/ml, micrograms per milliliter. INR, international normalized ratio.

Table 2-11 Normal values for enzymes

Enzyme	Normal Value	Significance
Aspartate aminotransferase (AST); formerly SGOT	6-18 U/L (women); 7-21 U/L (men)	Cellular damage in a variety of organs or tissues, including the heart, brain, liver, and skeletal muscle may result in the release of enzymes that can be measured in the serum. Isoenzymes help to more specifically identify where the damage has occurred. Cardiac isoenzymes are CK-MB, LDH_1, LDH_2.
Creatine kinase (CK)	96-140 U/L (women); 38-174 U/L (men)	
CK-MB	0%	
Lactic dehydrogenase (LDH)	90-200 U/L	
LDH_1	17.5%-28.3% of total LDH	
LDH_2	30.4%-36.4% of total LDH ($LDH_1 < LDH_2$)	

U/L, units per liter.

Table 2-12 **Enzyme changes with myocardial infarction**

Enzyme Elevated	Onset	Peak	Duration
AST	12-18 hr	24-48 hr	3-4 days
CK	4-6 hr	12-24 hr	3-4 days
CK-MB	4-6 hr	12-24 hr	2-3 days
LDH	24-48 hr	3-6 days	7-10 days
$LDH_1 > LDH_2$ (LDH flip)	12-24 hr	48 hr	Variable

Quick guide to arterial blood gas (ABG) interpretation

1. Evaluate pH

   Below 7.35—acidotic

   Above 7.45—alkalotic

   Normal—no acid-base imbalance or compensation has occurred

2. Evaluate Pco_2 (respiratory component)

   Above 45—respiratory acidosis or compensation for metabolic alkalosis

   Below 35—respiratory alkalosis or compensation for metabolic acidosis

   Normal—no respiratory component to the imbalance

3. Evaluate HCO_3 (metabolic component)

   Above 26—metabolic alkalosis or compensation for respiratory acidosis

   Below 22—metabolic acidosis or compensation for respiratory alkalosis

   Normal—no metabolic component to the imbalance

4. Determine cause and treatment of acid-base imbalance by evaluating other pertinent patient data

Oxyhemoglobin dissociation curve

The oxyhemoglobin dissociation curve depicts the relationship between the partial pressure of oxygen and the percent saturation of the hemoglobin. A small change in Pao_2 will significantly affect hemoglobin saturation in patients who are functioning on the steep portion of the curve (Figure 2-3). As the curve shifts to the right, hemoglobin and oxygen are less tightly bound, thus more oxygen is released to the cell. As the curve shifts to the left, hemoglobin and oxygen are more tightly bound, thus less oxygen is released to the cell.

Table 2-13 Hematology and associated cardiovascular implications

Test	Normal Value	Cardiovascular Implications
Hemoglobin/hematocrit	12-16 g/dl, 37%-47% (women); 14-18 g/dl, 40%-54% (men)	Low—cardiac work is increased as the heart compensates with increased heart rate and stroke volume; angina may result High—viscosity of the blood increases, thus increasing the risk for thromboembolic events
Myoglobin	30-90 ng/ml	Myoglobin is an oxygen-binding protein found in cardiac muscle and skeletal muscle High—associated with myocardial infarction and skeletal muscle injury

g/dl, grams per deciliter. ng/ml, nanograms per milliliter.

Table 2-14 Normal arterial and venous blood gases

	Arterial	Venous
pH	7.35-7.45	7.31-7.41
P_{CO_2}	35-45 mm Hg	41-51 mm Hg
HCO_3	22-26 mEq/L	22-26 mEq/L
P_{O_2}	80-100 mm Hg	35-45 mm Hg
O_2 saturation	95%	60-80%

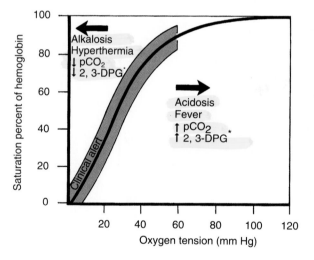

Figure 2-3
Oxyhemoglobin dissociation curve.

* 2,3-Diphosphoglycerate (inorganic phosphate found in red blood cells; increases with hypoxemia and anemia).

Table 2-15 **Acid/base imbalances**

Imbalance	ABG Values	Common Causes
Respiratory acidosis	pH low, PCO_2 high,* HCO_3 normal or high	Hypoventilation; drug overdose, use of anesthetics, chronic lung disease, sedation
Respiratory alkalosis	pH high, PCO_2 low,* HCO_3 normal, or low	Hyperventilation; anxiety, pain, mechanical ventilator, salicylates
Metabolic acidosis	pH low, PCO_2 low, HCO_3 low*	Hypoxia, renal failure, diarrhea, diabetic ketoacidosis, shock
Metabolic alkalosis	pH high, PCO_2 high, HCO_3 high*	Loss of gastrointestinal juices, potassium or chloride depletion, bicarbonate administration

*Primary abnormality.

Table 2-16 **Significance of changes in SvO_2**

SvO_2	Common Causes
Downward trend	*Decreased supply* caused by anemia, low cardiac output (dysrhythmias), decreased arterial oxygen saturation (suctioning)
	Increased demand caused by increased oxygen consumption (pain)
Upward trend	*Increased supply* caused by high cardiac output (sepsis), increased arterial oxygen saturation, blood transfusion.
	Decreased demand caused by less oxygen consumption by the tissues (hypothermia, cyanide toxicity)

Clinical Alert

· Arterial oxygen saturation (Sao_2) is monitored via blood gases and pulse oximetry (Spo_2)
· An $Sao_2 < 90$ equates with a Pao_2 in the 50s, a dangerous level for the patient.

Mixed venous oxygen saturation (Svo_2)

Svo_2 is the average percentage of hemoglobin bound with oxygen in venous blood and reflects overall tissue utilization of oxygen. Continuous monitoring can be used to assess oxygen supply balance. Changes in Svo_2 typically precede other indications of imbalance between oxygen supply and demand and thus can be a valuable monitoring parameter in the critically ill patient.

Normal values are 60% to 80%; the sample is obtained in the pulmonary artery where venous blood is mixed. See Table 2-16 for the significance of abnormal values.

Clinical Alert

If Svo_2 changes by $\pm$ 10% from baseline or drops below 60%, evaluate the patient to identify the cause of the supply demand imbalance and intervene appropriately.

Diagnostic Tests

Both invasive and noninvasive diagnostic tests are available to provide information about cardiovascular status. The data obtained can be used for numerous purposes including diagnosis, assessment of disease progression, and evaluation of treatment.

Electrocardiogram (ECG)

Purpose

A 12-lead ECG provides information on rate, rhythm, conduction, areas of ischemia and infarct, hypertrophy, axis, effect of cardiac drugs, effect of electrolyte imbalance, and pacemaker function (see Chapter 3 for information about pacemakers). One lead is used primarily for monitoring dysrhythmias.

ECG leads

A lead allows for recording the potential differences between two electrodes (one positive and one negative). As electrical activity of the heart moves in the direction of the positive electrode, a positive

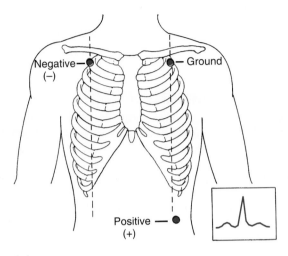

Figure 2-4
Lead II. Positive electrode—left leg; negative electrode—right arm.

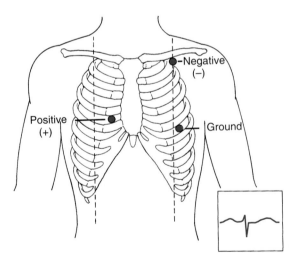

Figure 2-5
Lead MCL$_1$. Positive electrode—fourth intercostal space right of sternum; negative electrode—beneath left midclavicle.

or upright complex is seen on the ECG. As the electrical activity moves away from the positive electrode, a negative or downward complex is seen on the ECG. Common monitoring leads are leads II, MCL₁, and V₁ (Figures 2-4 to 2-6). More complete information is obtained from the 12-lead ECG, which includes six limb leads and six precordial leads (Figure 2-7).

Clinical Alert

· MCL₁ is helpful in differentiating ventricular ectopy from supraventricular ectopy with aberrant ventricular conduction (Table 2-17). It is also used to differentiate right and left bundle branch block (BBB). BBB exists when there is a normal PR with a QRS ≥ 0.12 second. If there is an rSR in MCL₁, RBBB is present; if the QRS is primarily negative in MCL₁, LBBB is present.

· The Lewis lead is less commonly used but may be helpful in enhancing visualization of P waves. The positive electrode is placed in the fourth intercostal space right of the sternum; the negative

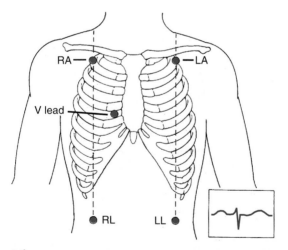

Figure 2-6
Lead V₁—five-lead system. V lead—fourth intercostal space right of sternum; LA lead—beneath left midclavicle; RA lead—beneath right midclavicle; LL lead—left abdomen; RL lead—right abdomen.

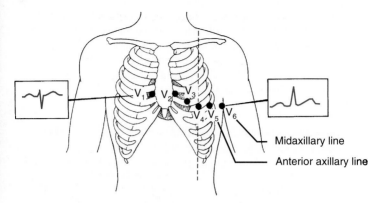

Figure 2-7
Precordial leads. V lead (positive) can be placed at identified locations to record $V_1, V_2, V_3, V_4, V_5,$ or V_6.

electrode is placed in the second intercostal space right of the sternum.

Basics for ECG interpretation

ECG paper is standardized (see Figure 2-8).
- Vertical lines measure time: small boxes represent 0.04 second, large boxes represent 0.20 second, markers at top of the paper are placed at 3-second intervals
- Horizontal lines measure voltage: small boxes (1 mm) represent 0.1 mV, large boxes (5 mm) represent 0.5 mV

Components of the ECG include the P, QRS, and T waves; occasionally a U wave may be present (see Figure 2-9). Normal timing for the various components can be found in Table 2-18.

Several methods are available to calculate heart rate (Figures 2-10 and 2-11). Three of these methods are:

1. Count the number of intervals between QRS complexes in a 6-second strip and multiply by 10.
2. Count the number of large boxes between two R waves and divide into 300.
3. Count the number of small boxes between two R waves and divide into 1500.

Table 2-17   **Aberrancy versus ventricular ectopy***

Favors Aberrancy	Favors Ventricular Ectopy
Triphasic QRS (i.e., rSR' in V_1)	QRS > 0.14 sec (no preexisting bundle branch block)
QRS 0.12-0.14 sec	AV dissociation (no relationship between P and QRS)
Identifiable P waves that bear a constant relationship to QRS	Concordant pattern (entirely positive or negative QRS in precordial leads)
	Absent RS complex in all precordial leads
	If QRS is positive in V_1
	· Monophasic or biphasic QRS in V_1
	· Taller left rabbit ear in V_1
	· R:S ratio in V_6 <1 (deep S)
	If QRS is negative in V_1
	· Broad R (>0.03 sec)
	· Slurred/notched S wave downstroke in V_1 or V_2
	· Delayed S wave nadir (onset of QRS to peak of S wave >0.06 sec) in V_1 or V_2
	· Any Q wave in V_6

*V_1 and MCL_1 are similar, thus MCL_1 is the preferred monitoring lead when trying to differentiate aberrancy from ectopy.

Table 2-18   **ECG components with normal timing**

Component	Normal Timing
P	0.06-0.11 sec
PR interval	0.12-0.20 sec
QRS	0.10 sec
T	0.16 sec
QT interval*	Varies with heart rate; usually 0.35-0.44 sec with heart rates of 60-100
U	Variable

*QTc (QT corrected for heart rate) $= \dfrac{QT}{\sqrt{RR}}$ interval; normal ≤ 0.39 second (men); ≤ 0.44 second (women).

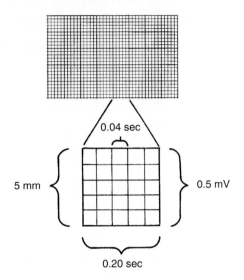

0.04 sec

5 mm

0.5 mV

0.20 sec

Figure 2-8
ECG grid.

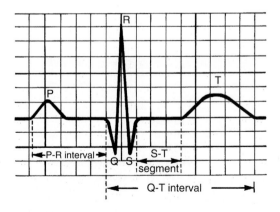

Figure 2-9
ECG complex.

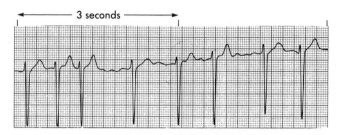

Figure 2-10
Rate calculation using Method 1. Use this method if rhythm is irregular. Count the number of intervals between QRS complexes in a 6-second strip and multiply by 10 (10 × 6 seconds = 60 seconds or 1 minute). Estimated rate is 80 beats/minute.

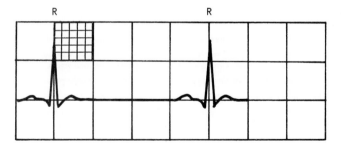

Figure 2-11
Rate calculations using Methods 2 and 3. Method 2: Count the number of large boxes between two R waves and divide into 300 (300 ÷ 4 large boxes = 75 beats/minute). Method 3: Count the number of small boxes between two R waves and divide into 1500 (1500 ÷ 20 small boxes = 75 beats/minute).

Clinical Alert

If the rhythm is irregular, use method 1. The rate will be an estimate.

Rhythm strip analysis

Specific steps for analysis of a rhythm strip are presented in the
box below.

Analysis of a Rhythm Strip

---

1. Calculate rate—atrial and ventricular
2. Note rhythm—regular, irregular
3. Identify P waves—note relationship to QRS, configura-
   tion
4. Determine PR interval
5. Determine QRS interval
6. Determine QT interval
7. Identify dysrhythmia, if possible
8. Identify possible implications for the patient

Inherent in analysis of a rhythm strip is consideration of the he-
modynamics and predictive aspects of the rhythm. Rhythms that
originate above the ventricles (supraventricular) generally have less
of an adverse effect on cardiac output than those that originate in
the ventricles. Rhythms such as pulseless ventricular tachycardia,
ventricular fibrillation, and asystole have a profound effect on cardiac output and represent emergency situations that require cardiopulmonary resuscitation (CPR).

Typically, supraventricular rhythms can be differentiated from
those of ventricular origin on the basis of QRS duration or width:
QRS ≤ 0.10 second (narrow QRS) indicates supraventricular origin; QRS ≥ 0.12 second (wide QRS) indicates ventricular origin.
Occasionally, however, a supraventricular beat may be temporarily
conducted through the ventricle in an abnormal or aberrant manner,

producing a wide QRS. Criteria for differentiating supraventricular beats conducted aberrantly from ventricular ectopy can be found in Table 2-17. The distinction is important clinically because treatment for ventricular ectopy is different from that for a supraventricular tachycardia, as discussed later in this chapter.

Heart rate also affects cardiac output (cardiac output = heart rate × stroke volume). Adverse effects of fast rates include increase in myocardial oxygen consumption (demand), decrease in diastolic filling time, and decrease in cardiac output (supply). The major adverse effect of a slow rate is a decrease in cardiac output.

Also of importance to cardiac output are atrioventricular (AV) synchrony and the contribution of atrial contraction to ventricular filling. AV dissociation resulting from ventricular tachycardia, complete heart block, or atrial fibrillation causes loss of effective atrial contraction. This in turn may decrease cardiac output 15% to 30%.

Rhythms that initially have no hemodynamic significance may become more serious rhythm disturbances that do adversely affect cardiac output. For example, frequent premature atrial contractions may be the forerunner of atrial fibrillation, premature ventricular contractions may precede ventricular tachycardia or ventricular fibrillation, and Mobitz type II heart block frequently progresses to complete heart block. An awareness of the possible progression of a dysrhythmia can minimize complications and result in more timely intervention.

Clinical Alert

· Monitor for signs and symptoms of decreased cardiac output (see Appendix C).
· Evaluate pain status.
· Be aware of predisposing factors for dysrhythmias: electrolyte imbalance, hypokalemia, hypoxia, pain, anemia, hypovolemia, hypotension, and digitalis toxicity.
· A prolonged QT may lead to a life-threatening dysrhythmia known as torsades de pointes or polymorphic ventricular tachycardia. Hypokalemia, hypocalcemia and drugs such as quinidine and procainamide prolong the QT interval.

Common dysrhythmias with major variances from normal sinus rhythm

Refer to Chapter 4 for specific drug information.

Sinus bradycardia

Rate	Rhythm	Major Variance
Atrial: < 60	Regular	Slow rate
Venltricular: < 60	Regular	

Treatment: None, if no evidence of decreased cardiac output (i.e., hypotension, chest pain, dizziness). Atropine, if symptomatic.

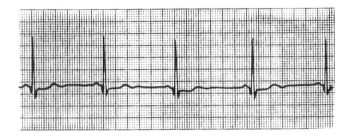

Sinus tachycardia

Rate	Rhythm	Major Variance
Atrial: > 100	Regular	Fast rate
Ventricular: > 100	Regular	

Treatment: None: investigate cause. Causes include sympathetic stimulation, emotional reactions, hypotension, fever, hypoxia, and vagolytic and sympathomimetic drugs.

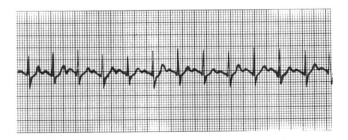

Sinus arrhythmia

Rate	Rhythm	Major Variance
Increases with inspiration, decreases with expiration	Irregular	Irregularity, variable rate

Treatment: None.

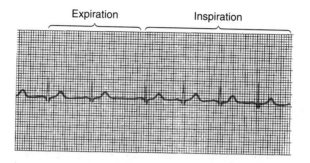

Premature atrial complex (PAC)

Rate	Rhythm	Major Variance
Determined by underlying rhythm	Irregular because of PAC	P of PAC is premature and a different shape than the sinus P

Treatment: None if infrequent. If frequent, omit irritants such as caffeine and nicotine. Drugs such as digoxin, quinidine, or procainamide (Pronestyl) may be used.

PAC

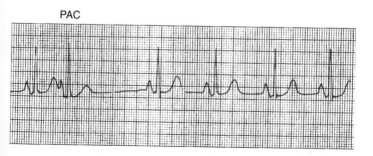

*Atrial tachycardia (with block)**

Rate	Rhythm	Major Variance
Atrial: 140-250	Regular	Fast atrial rate; loss of 1:1 AV conduction
Ventricular: depends on AV conduction ratio	Regular	When 1:1 AV conduction is present, both atrial and ventricular rates are fast.

Treatment: Identify and treat cause. Frequently associated with digitalis toxicity.

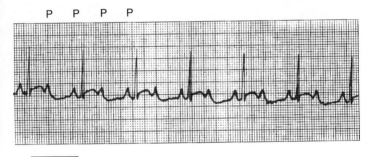

*Without block a QRS follows each P wave

Atrial flutter

Rate	Rhythm	Major Variance
Atrial: 250-300	Regular	Sawtooth pattern of flutter waves, fast rate
Ventricular: 125-150; depends on AV conduction	Regular/irregular	

Treatment: Digitalis, diltiazem (Cardizem), verapamil (Calan, Isoptin), quinidine, propranolol (Inderal), cardioversion (if hemodynamically unstable).

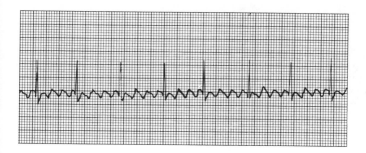

Atrial fibrillation

Rate	Rhythm	Major Variance
Atrial: > 350	Irregular	Fibrillatory waves instead of P waves, no pattern to irregularity
Ventricular: 110-180 (uncontrolled); < 100 (controlled)	Irregular	

Treatment: Digitalis, diltiazem (Cardizem), verapamil (Calan, Isoptin), quinidine, propranolol (Inderal), cardioversion (if hemodynamically unstable).

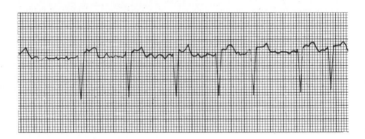

Accelerated idiojunctional rhythm

Rate	Rhythm	Major Variance
Atrial: unable to determine	Regular	Loss of AV synchrony, loss of normal P wave
Ventricular: 60-100	Regular	

Treatment: Identify and treat the cause.

Paroxysmal supraventricular tachycardia (PSVT)

Rate	Rhythm	Major Variance
Atrial: unable to determine	Regular	Rapid rate that begins and ends abruptly
Ventricular: 170-250	Regular	

Treatment: Vagal maneuvers, adenosine (Adenocard), verapamil (Calan, Isoptin), propranolol (Inderal), cardioversion (if hemodynamically unstable).

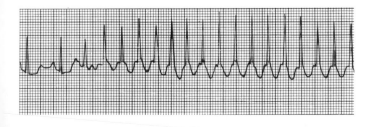

Premature ventricular complex (PVC)

Rate	Rhythm	Major Variance
Determined by underlying rhythm	Irregular due to PVC	No P wave; bizarre, broad QRS that is premature; T wave opposite deflection of QRS

Treatment: Lidocaine, procainamide (Pronestyl) (see below)

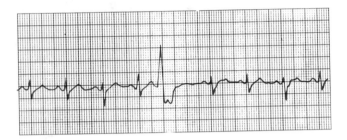

Criteria for Treatment of PVCs

Paired
Multifocal
> 6 per minute
R on T

Ventricular tachycardia (VT)

Rate	Rhythm	Major Variance
Atrial: variable	Usually regular	Broad QRS, fast rate, AV dissociation
Ventricular: 100-170	Usually regular	

Treatment: Lidocaine, procainamide (Pronestyl), cardioversion (if hemodynamically unstable). If pulseless, treat as ventricular fibrillation.

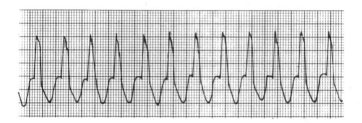

Ventricular fibrillation (VF)

Rate	Rhythm	Major Variance
Unable to determine	Chaotic	Bizarre, erratic activity without QRS complexes

Treatment: CPR, defibrillation, lidocaine, bretylium tosylate (Bretylol).

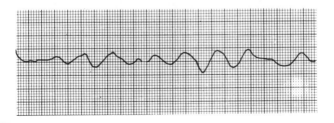

Torsades de pointes

Rate	Rhythm	Major Variance
Atrial: unable to determine		Phasic variation in polarity of QRS
Ventricular: 150-250	Regular/irregular	

Treatment: Identify the cause; temporary overdrive pacing, magnesium sulfate.

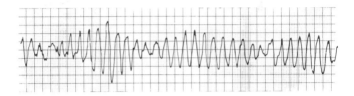

First-degree atrioventricular block

Rate	Rhythm	Major Variance
Atrial: 60-100	Regular	PR interval > 0.20 sec
Ventricular: 60-100	Regular	

Treatment: None.

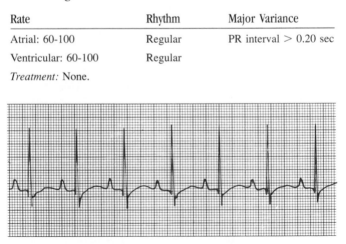

Second-degree atrioventricular block, Mobitz type I (Wenckebach)

Rate	Rhythm	Major Variance
Atrial: 60-100	Regular	Lengthening PR, shortening RR, pauses that are less than twice the shortest cycle
Ventricular: less than atrial	Irregular	Some P waves not followed by QRS

Treatment: None.

PR.28   PR.38   PR.40

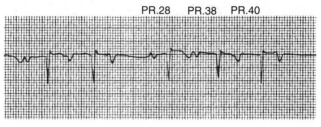

Second-degree atrioventricular block, Mobitz type II

Rate	Rhythm	Major Variance
Atrial: 60-100	Regular	Constant PR interval
Ventricular: less than atrial	Irregular	Some P waves not followed by QRS

Treatment: Atropine, pacemaker.

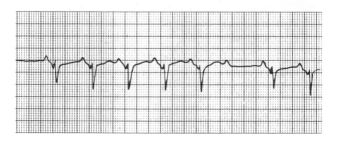

Third-degree atrioventricular block (complete AV block)

Rate	Rhythm	Major Variance
Atrial: 60-100	Regular	Variable PR interval; no relationship between P and QRS
Ventricular: < 58	Regular	Slow ventricular rate

Treatment: Pacemaker.

Select ECG changes

Hypothermia, electrolyte abnormalities, and various drugs may cause ECG changes. Changes on the 12-lead ECG also depict the evolution and location of myocardial infarction (Tables 2-19 and 2-20). Axis deviation may be responsible for certain other ECG changes. Figure 2-12 identifies a quick two-lead system for determining electrical axis, and Table 2-21 lists common causes of axis deviation.

Clinical Alert

· ST segment elevation of > 1 mm in V_4R (right precordial lead in V_4 position) has high predictive value for right ventricular infarction.
· Other conditions that can affect the ECG include:
  Ischemia (fixed lesion)—ST segment depression
  Ischemia (coronary vasospasm)—ST segment elevation
  Atrial abnormality/enlargement—changes in P wave duration and contour (Table 2-22)

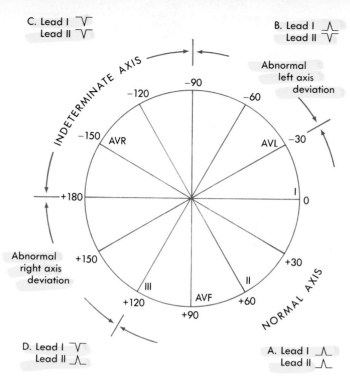

Figure 2-12

Axis determination using leads I and II. Evaluation of the QRS in leads I and II provides a quick method for estimating axis. **A,** If the QRS is upright in both leads I and II, the axis is normal. **B,** If the QRS is upright in lead I and down in lead II, left axis deviation is present. **C,** If the QRS is down in both leads I and II, indeterminate axis is present. **D,** If the QRS is down in lead I and upright in lead II, right axis deviation is present.

Table 2-19 Evolutionary changes of myocardial infarction

Change	Significance	Onset	Duration
T wave inversion	Ischemia	6-24 hr	Months to years
ST elevation	Injury	Immediate	1-6 weeks
Q waves (0.04 sec wide and/or 25% of R wave amplitude)	Necrosis	Immediate to several days	Generally permanent

Table 2-20   **Types of infarctions**

Anatomic Location	ECG Patterns
Lateral	I, aVL, V_5, V_6; abnormal Q wave, ST elevation, T wave inversion
Inferior	II, III, aVF; abnormal Q wave, ST elevation, T wave inversion
Anterior	V_1, V_2, V_3, V_4; abnormal Q wave, loss of R wave progression, ST elevation, T wave inversion
Posterior	V_1, V_2; tall R wave, ST depression, tall symmetrical T wave

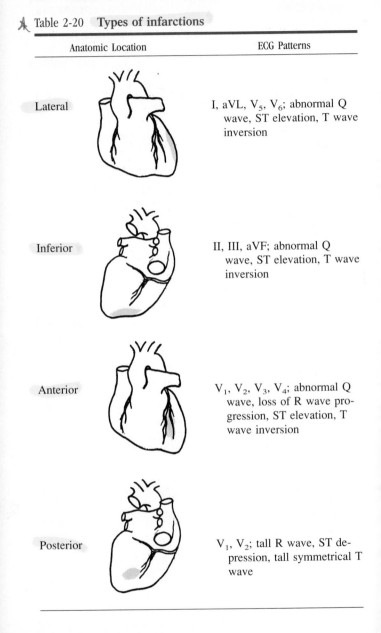

Table 2-21   Causes of axis deviation

Left Axis Deviation	Right Axis Deviation
Normal variant	Normal variant
Left anterior hemiblock (LAHB)	Left posterior hemiblock (LPHB)
Left bundle branch block (LBBB)	Right ventricular hypertrophy (RVH)
Left ventricular hypertrophy (LVH)	Limb lead reversal
Obesity	Dextrocardia
	Childhood
Inferior myocardial infarction	Lateral myocardial infarction

Table 2-22   Chamber enlargement

Chamber	Changes
RA	Tall, peaked P wave (> 2.5 mm) in II, III, aVF; low or isoelectric P wave in I; P waves in V_1, V_2 may be upright with increased amplitude
LA	P wave duration > 0.12 sec, P wave notched and upright in I, II, V_4 to V_6; wide, deep, negative component to P wave in V_1
RV	Right axis deviation, R/S ratio > 1 in V_1; ST segment depression and T wave inversion in V_1 and sometimes in V_2; late intrinsicoid deflection in V_1 or V_2
LV*	Increased voltage: R or S wave in limb leads ≥ 20 mm or S wave in V_1 or $V_2 \geq 30$ mm or R wave in V_5 or $V_6 \geq 30$ mm, 3 points ST changes: with digitalis, 1 point; without digitalis, 2 points LA enlargement, 3 points Left axis deviation, 2 points (-30 or more) QRS duration > 0.09 second, 1 point Intrinsicoid deflection in V_5 or $V_6 > 0.05$ second, 1 point

*4 points, LVH likely; 5 points, LVH present.

Ventricular hypertrophy—increased QRS amplitude, delayed intrinsicoid deflection (time to reach peak of R wave), changes in ST segment, T wave, and axis. A point system has been developed to aid in the diagnosis of left ventricular hypertrophy (Table 2-22)
· Continuous ST segment monitoring in select leads assists in early identification of the location of ischemia/infarction.

Exercise Stress Testing (Treadmill, Graded Exercise Test, GEX)

Purpose

· Screen for ischemic heart disease
· Evaluate dysrhythmias
· Assess functional capacity and cardiac reserve

Description

The exercise stress test combines ECG with exercise test to observe, measure, and record physiologic response to a known amount of work. Patient walks on the treadmill until becoming symptomatic, until target heart rate is achieved, or until the technician determines the test should be terminated.

Ischemic response is 1 mm or more flat or downsloping ST segment depression that lasts 0.08 second or longer. The examination time is 1 to 1½ hours.

Patient preparation

Explain the procedure and obtain signed consent. The patient should have no food, coffee, or cigarettes before the test; water is allowed. The patient should wear loose clothing and comfortable shoes. The physician may elect to discontinue some medications prior to testing. Obtain baseline vital signs.

Post test

Monitor vital signs and ECG until vital signs return to the baseline level.

Echocardiography (M-mode, two dimensional, transesophageal)

Purpose

· Identify structural abnormalities, such as chamber enlargement, ventricular or septal hypertrophy, valvular stenosis or insufficiency, intracardiac tumors or vegetations, abdominal aneurysm

- Identify effusion
- Evaluate valvular prosthesis
- Evaluate ventricular wall motion

Description

Echocardiography uses ultrasound to examine the size, shape, and motion of cardiac valves and chambers, and the size and shape of abdominal aorta. The patient lies on the left side or sits up leaning forward. There is no pain or discomfort. A hand-held transducer with conducting gel is placed on the chest or abdomen. A trans-esophageal echocardiogram (TEE) visualizes the heart via an endo-scope positioned in the esophagus. The examination time is 30 to 45 minutes.

Patient preparation

Explain the purpose of the test. For an abdominal echo, the patient should take nothing by mouth (except water) for 12 hours before the test. Schedule the test before a barium x-ray procedure.

A signed consent is necessary for a TEE, and the patient should take nothing by mouth for 4 to 6 hours before the test. Obtain base-line vital signs. Before inserting the endoscope, the physician will topically anesthetize the oropharynx and sedate the patient. Func-tional suctioning equipment should be readily available. Monitor vital signs, cardiac rhythm, and oxygen saturation (via oximetry) throughout the procedure.

Post test

No special monitoring is necessary following M-mode and two-di-mensional echocardiography. After the TEE test, monitor for evi-dence of oversedation and esophageal perforation (substernal pain, neck discomfort, thirst, increased pain with swallowing, tachycar-dia, upper abdominal rigidity, a "crunch" heard on auscultation over the sternum). The patient should take nothing by mouth for 30 to 60 minutes following the procedure because the topical anesthe-sia of the pharynx may impair swallowing.

Myocardial Blood Flow Evaluation (Thallium Scan, Cold Spot Imaging)

Purpose

Radioisotope studies are used to identify any area of stress-induced ischemia or an old infarct.

Description

This radioisotope study uses thallium 201, which concentrates in normal tissue but not in ischemic or infarcted tissue (i.e., a cold spot). It is often paired with an exercise test to evaluate myocardial blood flow with increased demand. Cold spots that reperfuse with rest indicate ischemia; cold spots that remain indicate infarct.

With an IV in place, the patient walks on the treadmill to a point determined by the physician. Thallium is administered IV and the patient walks an additional 30 to 60 seconds on the treadmill. The patient then lies down for scanning. A repeat scan may be done 4 hours later at rest to check for redistribution of thallium to the cold spot. The examination time is 2 hours.

Patient preparation

Explain the procedure to the patient and obtain signed consent. The patient should take nothing by mouth and should not smoke for 2 hours before the test. Obtain baseline vital signs.

Post test

Monitor vital signs and ECG until all return to baseline levels.

Myocardial Infarct Imaging (Hot Spot Imaging, Pyrophosphate Heart Scan)

Purpose

· Identify infarcted tissue 24 to 72 hours after a suspected myocardial infarction
· Helpful in differentiating old and new areas of infarct

Description

Myocardial infarct imaging uses technetium pyrophosphate, which concentrates in acutely necrotic myocardium (a hot spot). It begins to accumulate in necrotic tissue 12 to 16 hours after onset of infarct and peaks at 24 to 72 hours.

An IV injection of technetium is given, followed by a 30-minute to 3-hour waiting period while the isotope accumulates in necrotic heart muscle. The patient lies quietly on the examining table while the scanning is done. The examination time is 30 minutes.

Patient preparation

Explain the procedure to the patient.

Post test

Special monitoring related to the test is unnecessary.

Gated Blood Pool Scan (MUGA Multigated Acquisition Scan)

Purpose

· Evaluate wall motion
· Calculate ejection fraction, cardiac output, and end diastolic volume

Description

Gated blood pool scan uses technetium pyrophosphate to tag red blood cells. A computer is utilized to analyze ventricular function. The test may be performed with stress testing. An ejection fraction < 50% indicates ventricular dysfunction.

The patient is supine, technetium is injected IV, a scintillation camera records movement of the isotope through the heart. Exercise testing may also be performed. The examination time is 30 minutes.

Patient preparation

Explain the test to the patient. If a stress test is done, obtain signed consent. The patient should take nothing by mouth and should not smoke for 2 hours before the test. Obtain baseline vital signs.

Post test

If a stress test is done, monitor vital signs and ECG until all return to baseline.

Doppler Studies

Purpose

· Evaluate arterial and venous blood flow
· Obtain segmental leg pressures (arterial study)
· Monitor ankle/arm pressure before and after treadmill test (arterial study)
· Rule out presence of deep vein thrombosis (venous study)

Description

A Doppler study uses an ultrasound beam that is reflected off red blood cells. The frequency or pitch changes in proportion to the velocity of blood flow; the normal arterial pulse produces a pulsating and multiphasic signal. A wave tracing shows a prominent systolic component and one or more diastolic sounds. The normal venous sound is intermittent (resembling a windstorm) and is phasic with respiration.

Both the arterial and venous studies are done at rest to determine baseline values. The arterial study may also include walking on the treadmill.

To arrive at the ankle/arm index, divide ankle pressure by arm pressure. The index should be ≥ 1.0. Ankle pressure decreases with disease, thus the index falls below 1.0.

A hand-held transducer is used to obtain the various pressures. The examination time is 1 hour.

Patient preparation

Explain the test to the patient. If the test involves walking on the treadmill, obtain a signed consent. The patient should not smoke for 2 hours before walking on the treadmill. Obtain baseline vital signs. Note the presence or absence of peripheral pulses.

Post test

No special monitoring related to resting arterial or venous studies is necessary. If the treadmill is included with the arterial study, monitor vital signs and ECG until all return to baseline values.

Impedance Plethysmography (IPG)

Purpose

Impedance plethysmography is used to measure changes in venous volume suggestive of deep vein thrombosis.

Description

A blood pressure cuff is applied to the thigh and inflated to impede venous flow (about 45 to 50 mm Hg) but not arterial flow. Electrodes placed on the calf measure electrical resistance, which results from the changes in venous volume. With deep vein thrombosis, changes in venous volume will be less than expected.

The patient is supine with the test leg elevated 30° to 35°. The knee is flexed.

Examination time is 30 to 45 minutes.

Patient preparation

Explain the test to the patient.

Post test

This test requires no special monitoring.

Cardiac Catheterization (Right-Sided Heart Catheterization, Left-Sided Heart Catheterization, Coronary Arteriography, or Ventricular Angiography)

Purpose

- Identify blockage or spasm in coronary artery or bypass graft
- Measure pressures within chambers and great vessels
- Evaluate valve/ventricular function
- Provide access to coronary artery for percutaneous transluminal coronary angioplasty (PTCA), intracoronary streptokinase (Streptase) administration, atherectomy, laser therapy, insertion of stent
- Provide access to valve for percutaneous balloon valvuloplasty

Description

The catheter is introduced into the heart or coronary ostia; introduction of contrast media allows evaluation of the flow through coronary arteries and cardiac chambers.

The patient lies on an x-ray table and is awake during the procedure in order to follow the physician's instructions. When the contrast is injected, the patient may experience a warm, flushed sensation. Examination time is 1 to 2 hours.

Patient preparation

Explain the procedure to the patient and obtain signed consent. The patient should take nothing by mouth for 3 to 6 hours before the test (some physicians will order regular medications to be given with a sip of water). The patient may wear dentures during the procedure. No premedication is required, although some physicians may order diazepam (Valium). Obtain baseline vital signs and assess peripheral pulses. Explain the post-test routine.

Post test

Bedrest is necessary for 2 to 12 hours (depends on catheter insertion site). Monitor vital signs, check catheter insertion site for bleeding or swelling, do not flex affected extremity at catheter insertion site, check pulses distal to catheter insertion site, and encourage fluids.

Electrophysiology Study (EPS)

Purpose

The electrophysiology study is used to diagnose and evaluate the treatment of ventricular and supraventricular dysrhythmias, atrioventricular block, ventricular preexcitation, sick sinus syndrome, and syncope.

Description

Electrode catheters are inserted into the right side of the heart to measure resting electrical values; the heart is then paced to induce dysrhythmia. Under the controlled situation of the catheterization laboratory, effective ways of terminating the dysrhythmia can be evaluated.

The patient lies on the x-ray table during the procedure and may experience palpitations or racing of the heart when the heart is paced.

The examination time is 1 to 4 hours.

Patient preparation

Explain the procedure to the patient and obtain a signed consent. Discontinue antidysrhythmic drugs before the test as ordered by the physician. Nothing should be taken by mouth 3 to 6 hours before the test. The patient may wear dentures. Usually no premedication is ordered. If premedication is needed, diazepam (Valium) is the drug of choice because it produces no significant electrophysiologic effects. Obtain baseline vital signs and assess peripheral pulses. Explain the post test routine.

Post test

Monitoring is the same as that for cardiac catheterization.

Peripheral Arteriography

Purpose

· Identify area of blockage in vessel
· Identify location and size of aneurysm
· Provide access for angioplasty or thrombolytic therapy

Description

A catheter is introduced via the femoral artery, contrast medium is injected, and successive x-ray films are taken to evaluate the flow through specified vessel(s).

The patient lies on an x-ray table and may experience a warm, flushed feeling when the contrast is injected.

The examination time is 1 hour.

Patient preparation

Explain procedure to the patient and obtain signed consent. The patient should take nothing by mouth for 6 hours before the test. Obtain baseline vital signs. Note the presence or absence of peripheral pulses. Explain the post-test routine.

Post test

Bedrest is necessary for 6 to 8 hours. Keep the affected extremity straight, monitor vital signs, check catheter insertion site for bleeding or swelling, check pulses and circulation distal to the catheter insertion site, and encourage fluids.

Digital Subtraction Angiography (DSA)

Purpose

- Detect peripheral artery disease
- Aid postoperative evaluation of vascular surgery, such as arterial grafts

Description

Contrast is injected via a vein (brachial, femoral); with use of an image-intensifier video system, vessels are displayed on a monitor; by computer, the images not required are subtracted so the image of the desired vessel is heightened. There is less risk than in arteriography because the contrast is injected into a vein and 50% to 75% less contrast is required.

The patient lies on an x-ray table, initial x-rays are taken, a catheter is inserted into the selected vein, contrast is administered, and a second series of x-rays is taken.

The examination time is 30 to 45 minutes.

Patient preparation

Explain the procedure to the patient and obtain signed consent. The patient should take nothing by mouth for 2 hours before the test. Explain the post-test routine.

Post test

Check vital signs, observe the catheter insertion site, and encourage fluids.

Venography

Purpose

· Confirm the presence of deep vein thrombosis
· Assess deep vein valvular competence
· Evaluate congenital venous malformations

Description

Contrast medium is injected through the dorsal foot vein; x-ray films are taken to evaluate flow through the veins.

The patient lies on an x-ray table, an IV is introduced in the dorsal foot vein, contrast is injected, films are taken. The patient may experience transient burning when the contrast is injected. After x-rays are taken, the leg is elevated and normal saline is used to flush contrast through veins.

The examination time is 30 to 45 minutes.

Patient preparation

Explain the procedure to the patient and obtain signed consent. The patient may have only clear liquids for 4 hours before the test. Explain the post-test routine.

Post test

Monitor vital signs and check the catheter insertion site for bleeding and hematoma.

Clinical Alert

· Monitor for complications of the procedure: vascular damage, hemorrhage, thromboembolism, dysrhythmias, ischemia or infarction.
· Notify the physician immediately if the following occurs: diminished or absent pulses, bleeding that does not stop with pressure, change in vital signs, change in mentation.
· Be aware of complications such as cardiac failure, allergic reactions, seizures, and renal failure associated with contrast agents. Contrast medium is hypertonic, thus fluid status must be monitored closely. Since contrast medium is excreted by the kidneys, its hypertonic effect will be increased and prolonged by dehydration and/or poor renal function. Note BUN before and after the procedure.

Selected bibliography

Alspach J, editor: *Core curriculum for critical care nursing,* Philadelphia, 1991, Saunders.

American Nurses' Association, Division on Medical-Surgical Nursing Practice and American Heart Association Council on Cardiovascular Nursing: *Standards of cardiovascular nursing practice,* Kansas City, 1981, American Nurses' Association.

Apple S, Thurkauf G: Preparing for and understanding transesophageal echocardiography, *Crit Care Nurse* 12(6):29-34, 1992.

Braunwald E, editor: *Heart disease: a textbook of cardiovascular medicine,* Philadelphia, 1992, Saunders.

Conover M: *Pocket nurse guide to electrocardiography,* St Louis, 1990, Mosby.

Conover M: *Understanding electrocardiography,* St Louis, 1992, Mosby.

Drew B: Bedside electrocardiographic monitoring: state of the art for the 1990s, *Heart Lung* 20(6):610-623, 1991.

Guzzetta C, Dossey B: *Cardiovascular nursing: holistic practice,* St Louis, 1992, Mosby.

Hurst JW, editor: *The heart, arteries, and veins,* St Louis, 1990, McGraw-Hill.

Pagana K, Pagana T: *Mosby's diagnostic and laboratory test reference,* St Louis, 1992, Mosby.

Proulx R, et al: Detection of right ventricular myocardial infarction in patients with inferior wall myocardial infarction, *Crit Care Nurse* 12(5):50-59, 1992.

Textbook of advanced cardiac life support, Dallas, 1990, American Heart Association.

Tilkian AG, Conover MB: *Understanding heart sounds and murmurs,* Philadelphia, 1984, Saunders.

Procedures and Specialized Equipment

3

Hemodynamic Monitoring

Hemodynamic monitoring involves the measurement of pressures (arterial, venous, pulmonary artery, left atrial) to assess cardiovascular performance.

General Clinical Guidelines Related to Hemodynamic Monitoring

- Maintain 300 mm Hg continual pressure around flush solution bag.
- Use normal saline rather than D_5W for flush solution to minimize bacterial growth.
- Place transducer at phlebostatic axis prior to obtaining each pressure (Figure 3-1). The phlebostatic axis, a reference for identifying right atrial level, is the intersection of two imaginary lines—one drawn in the fourth intercostal space from the sternum to the side of the chest, the other drawn midway between the anterior and posterior chest. Accurate readings can be obtained with the head of the bed elevated up to 45°. Bed position does not alter accuracy of arterial pressures.
- Zero and calibrate the equipment once during each shift or if accuracy of readings is questionable.
- Take readings at end expiration (CVP, PA, PAWP).
- If the patient is on a mechanical ventilator, especially with PEEP or CPAP, true pressure readings may be altered. However, removal from the ventilator is generally not recommended.
- Pressure trends, rather than an isolated measurement, provide more reliable information.

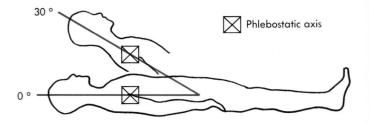

Figure 3-1
Phlebostatic axis, located at the fourth intercostal space mid anteroposterior chest. Reference for positioning the transducer at right atrial level.

· Check catheter position with a chest x-ray following insertion of CVP or PA catheter.
· Follow hospital policy regarding change of solution, tubing, dressing, catheter, and site. Recommended changes include the following:

> IV tubing—every 72 hours
> IV solution—every 24 hours
> Dressing—gauze, every 48 hours
> Catheter and site—every 3 to 4 days or with evidence of infection

· Follow electrical safety precautions:

> Ground bed and all electrical equipment
> Remove unnecessary electrical equipment from room
> Keep patient as dry as possible (change linens for diaphoresis, incontinence)
> Protect catheter from moisture
> Be sure hands are dry before contact with electrical equipment
> If patient has personal electrical equipment, such as a radio or razor, have it checked by a biomedical engineer before use.

Central Venous Pressure (CVP)

Description

CVP reflects pressure in the right atrium and systemic veins.

Normal values

0-8 mm Hg; 2-12 cm H_2O (see conversion table in Appendix D)

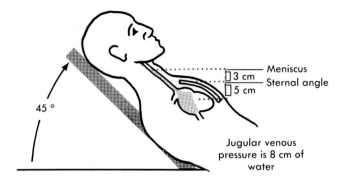

Figure 3-2
Estimation of central venous pressure.

Abnormal values

↓ CVP—hypovolemia, venodilatation from sepsis, drugs such as nitrates
↑ CVP—right ventricular failure, circulatory overload, cardiac tamponade, PEEP, chronic left ventricular failure

Measurement

Indirect

Use the sternal angle as reference, since in all positions the sternal angle remains 5 cm above mid–right atrial level (Figure 3-2). Identify the highest level of pulsations in internal jugular vein (meniscus). Determine the vertical distance in centimeters between the sternal angle and meniscus. Add that distance to the constant of 5 cm. An alternate method for estimating CVP uses the dorsal veins of the hand. With the patient seated, place one arm in a dependent position. Raise the arm slowly. Note the point at which the dorsal veins of the hand collapse. In a patient with normal venous pressure, the veins collapse at the point just above the sternal angle.

Direct

A manometer or transducer is used. Accuracy of measurement depends on several factors, including calibration of equipment and transducer position. A central line is placed with the catheter tip at the junction of the superior vena cava and right atrium, or a flow-directed pulmonary artery (PA) catheter is placed with the proximal lumen opening at the junction of the superior vena cava and right atrium. In addition to measuring CVP, a central or PA line can be used to:

- Administer fluids, blood, or blood products
- Administer total parenteral nutrition
- Administer incompatible drugs simultaneously
- Withdraw venous blood samples
- Phlebotomize the patient

Clinical Alert

When using a PA catheter, return monitor to PA waveform for continuous monitoring after CVP has been obtained. See General Clinical Guidelines Related to Hemodynamic Monitoring earlier in this chapter.

Pulmonary Artery Pressure (PAP)

Description

PAP reflects left-sided and right-sided heart pressures; pulmonary artery systolic (PAS) reflects the right ventricular pressure, pulmonary artery diastolic (PAD) and pulmonary artery wedge pressure (PAWP) reflect pressure in the left ventricle at end diastole (in the presence of a normal mitral valve with no pulmonary disease). See Figure 3-3 for waveforms and pressures at the time of insertion.

Normal values

Right atrium (RA) 0-8 mm Hg
Right ventricle (RV)
  Systolic 15-28 mm Hg
  Diastolic 0-8 mm Hg
PAS 15-30 mm Hg
PAD* 5-15 mm Hg
PA (mean) 10-20 mm Hg
PAWP* 4-12 mm Hg

Abnormal values

↑ PAS—right ventricular failure, constrictive pericarditis, cardiac tamponade, congestive failure, pulmonary hypertension
↑ PAD—left ventricular failure, mitral stenosis, pulmonary hypertension, left to right shunts

---

*Normally, PAD is 1 to 3 mm Hg higher than PAWP.

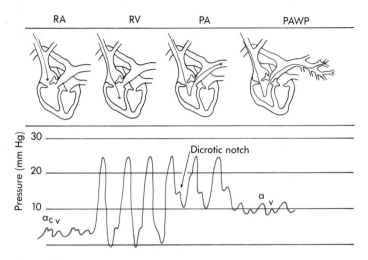

Figure 3-3
Waveforms and pressures with a flow-directed pulmonary artery catheter. *RA,* Right atrium; *RV,* right ventricle; *PA,* pulmonary artery; *PAWP,* pulmonary artery wedge pressure; *a wave,* atrial contraction; *c wave,* tricuspid closure; *v wave,* atrial filling; *dicrotic notch,* closure of pulmonic valve.

↑ PAWP—left ventricular failure, constrictive pericarditis, mitral valve dysfunction, fluid overload
↓ PAWP—hypovolemia, afterload reduction
A PAD 4 to 5 mm Hg > PAWP indicates increased pulmonary vascular resistance; a PAWP > PAD indicates overwedging or improper identification of PAD.

Measurement

A multilumen catheter is used. Complications of pulmonary artery catheters are listed in the box on p. 135. Accuracy of measurement depends on several variables, including calibration of equipment and transducer position. PAS, PAD, and mean PA are obtained from the monitor with the balloon deflated. To determine PAWP, slowly inject air into the balloon while simultaneously watching the monitor for a wedge waveform. Do not exceed balloon capacity indicated on the catheter, usually 1.5 cc. Stop inject-

Complications of Pulmonary Artery Catheters

Pulmonary embolism	Dysrhythmias
Damage to tricuspid valve	Intracardiac knotting of
Thrombophlebitis	catheter
Balloon rupture	Infection
Pulmonary infarction	Rupture of pulmonary
	artery

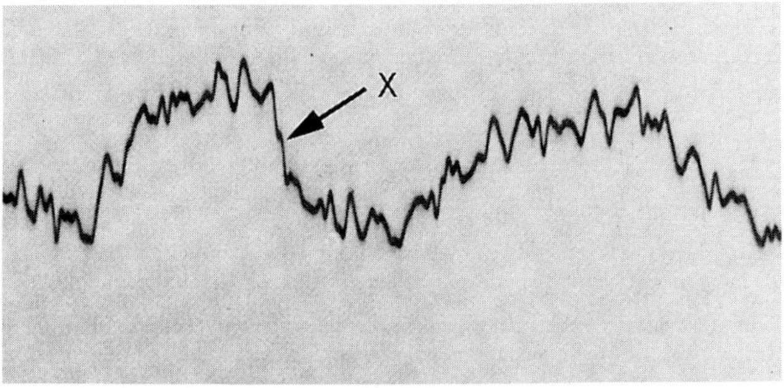

Figure 3-4
Identification of pulmonary artery wedge pressure. Respiratory variation in a patient breathing spontaneously. Read PAWP at X (end expiration).
From Daily E, Schroeder J: *Hemodynamic waveforms,* St Louis, 1990, Mosby.

ing air as soon as the wedge waveform is seen. After obtaining the wedge pressure, remove the syringe and allow the balloon to deflate passively. Watch monitor for return of PA waveform. All pressures are obtained at end expiration (Figure 3-4). The expiratory phase will differ depending on whether the patient is breathing spontaneously or with the aid of a ventilator. If the patient is breathing spontaneously, pressure decreases on inspiration and increases on expiration. If the patient is breathing with the aid of a ventilator, pressure increases on inspiration and decreases on expiration.

In addition to obtaining PA pressures, other uses for a PA catheter include:

Fluid and medication administration

Electrical pacing of the heart

Intermittent or continuous SvO_2 monitoring

Cardiac output, systemic vascular resistance (SVR), and pulmonary vascular resistance (PVR) calculation

To determine cardiac output, attach the thermistor port to the cardiac output computer. A specified amount of sterile fluid (usually 10 ml of normal saline) is rapidly injected (4 seconds or less) into the proximal port of the catheter. The computer calculates cardiac output. Generally, three consecutive measurements are obtained and averaged to determine cardiac output. Additional data that may be calculated include cardiac index, PVR, and SVR. (See Appendix B for formulas.) Cardiac index is cardiac output adjusted for body size. As cardiac index falls, tissue perfusion decreases. A cardiac index of 1.8 to 2.2 $L/min/m^2$ is consistent with hypoperfusion; < 1.8 $L/min/m^2$ is consistent with cardiogenic shock. Increased PVR represents increased work for the right ventricle; increased SVR represents increased work for the left ventricle.

Clinical Alert

· The balloon should not remain inflated in occluded position beyond 15 seconds or 2 to 3 respiratory cycles.
· If spontaneous wedging occurs, immediately notify physician to reposition the catheter. Turning the patient and/or having the patient cough may also be temporarily successful in changing catheter position.
· If PAD and PAWP are the same, monitor PAD pressures rather than repeatedly inflating the balloon for a PAWP.
· See General Clinical Guidelines related to Hemodynamic Monitoring earlier in this chapter.

Left Atrial Pressure (LAP)

Description

LAP is determined by direct measurement of pressure in the left atrium; it reflects left ventricular end diastolic pressure in the presence of a normal mitral valve. The left atrial waveform will be similar to that of the PAWP (see p. 134).

Normal values

4-12 mm Hg

Abnormal values

↑ LAP—mitral valve disease, left ventricular failure, volume overload, constrictive pericarditis, increased systemic vascular resistance

↓ LAP—hypovolemia, afterload reduction

Measurement

A catheter is placed in the left atrium at the time of heart surgery. The catheter is connected to a transducer for a continuous display of LAP; monitor LAP on "mean." Accuracy of measurement depends on several variables, including calibration of equipment and transducer position.

Clinical Alert

· An LA line provides a direct path for the entry of air or clots into the left heart, thus increasing the risk for systemic emboli. If the waveform dampens, aspirate until blood (and no air) is seen. If a blood return cannot be obtained or air is in the line, do not flush.

· See General Clinical Guidelines Related to Hemodynamic Monitoring earlier in this chapter.

Arterial Pressure

Description

Arterial pressure is determined by measuring systemic diastolic and systolic blood pressures.

Normal values

Systolic pressure—100-140 mm Hg
Diastolic pressure—60-90 mm Hg
Mean pressure (MAP)—70-105 mm Hg
(See Appendix B)

Measurement

Indirect

Use the proper-size blood pressure cuff (see p. 75) to obtain an accurate measurement. See the boxes on p. 138 that describe the procedures for obtaining an accurate blood pressure and the determination of pulsus paradoxus.

Direct

A catheter is placed in the radial, brachial, or femoral artery. The catheter is connected to a transducer with a continuous flush system. Accuracy of measurement depends on several variables, in-

Manual Determination of Cuff Blood Pressure

- Palpate pulse, inflate cuff to 30 mm above the point at which the pulse disappears.
- Deflate cuff at a rate of 2-3 mm Hg per second until the pulse is detected. This is the palpatory systolic pressure.
- Apply stethoscope over the artery and inflate cuff to 30 mm Hg above the palpatory systolic pressure.
- Deflate cuff at a rate of 2-3 mm Hg per second and note the changes in arterial sounds. The initial sound is the systolic pressure and the muffling or disappearance of sounds is the diastolic pressure.
- Auscultate until cuff pressure is zero.
- Wait 2 minutes before rechecking a blood pressure. Otherwise, a falsely elevated diastolic pressure may be obtained.
- NOTE: The silent interval between sounds is called the auscultatory gap. If the palpatory systolic pressure is not determined before the auscultatory pressure, cuff inflation may be stopped in the "silent" gap. When the cuff is deflated, the first sound heard may be the bottom of the auscultatory gap instead of the true systolic pressure.

Determination of Pulsus Paradoxus With a Blood Pressure Cuff

- Inflate cuff above known systolic pressure
- Have patient breathe normally
- Slowly deflate cuff, noting when the first sounds are heard
- Continue to deflate cuff (you may hear no sounds)
- Note when sounds begin again and are heard continuously
- Continue to deflate cuff until sounds muffle and disappear
- The difference between the first sound and continuous sounds is the pulsus paradoxus; >10 mm Hg is considered abnormal

cluding calibration of equipment and transducer position. (See Figure 3-5 for the normal arterial waveform and Table 3-1 for variations and their significance.) In addition to monitoring arterial pressure and waveform, an arterial catheter can also be used to obtain arterial blood samples.

Table 3-1 Variations in the arterial waveform (normal waveform: see Figure 3-5)

Variation	Waveform	
Corrigan's pulse (waterhammer pulse)		Associated with increased stroke volume (i.e., aortic insufficiency, anemia, or early hypovolemia)
Pulsus parvus		Associated with decreased stroke volume (i.e., left ventricular failure, or severe aortic stenosis)
Pulsus alternans		Associated with left ventricular failure and severe myocardial disease
Pulsus bigeminus		Associated with dysrhythmias that occur every other beat (i.e., PVCs)

Continued.

Table 3-1 Variations in the arterial waveform—cont'd

Variation		Waveform
Pulsus paradoxus (see box on p. 138)		Associated with hypovolemia or increased pooling in the pulmonary vasculature (i.e., tamponade)
Pulsus bisferiens (bisfid pulse)		Associated with hypertrophic cardiomyopathy (with obstruction) and severe anxiety states

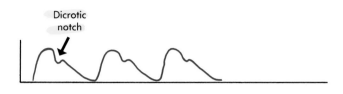

Figure 3-5
Normal arterial waveform. Dicrotic notch represents closure of aortic valve.

Clinical Alert

- Assure adequacy of collateral circulation before catheter insertion. Before attempting radial artery cannulation, perform the Allen test (Figure 3-6).
- Assess perfusion distal to catheter insertion site.
- After removal of the catheter, maintain pressure for 5 to 15 minutes, or until hemostasis is obtained.
- See General Clinical Guidelines Related to Hemodynamic Monitoring earlier in this chapter.

Troubleshooting Hemodynamic Monitoring Systems

A variety of problems may be encountered while monitoring hemodynamic parameters. Table 3-2 summarizes common problems, causes, and possible solutions.

Specialized Equipment

The availability of specialized equipment has greatly enhanced the ability to care for patients with cardiovascular disease. Despite complications, devices such as defibrillators, pacemakers, and the intra-aortic balloon pump have saved many lives.

Intra-Aortic Balloon Pump (IABP)
Description

The intra-aortic balloon pump (IABP) is a mechanical assist device consisting of a balloon positioned in the descending thoracic aorta that augments diastolic pressure and decreases afterload for the left ventricle (Figure 3-7).

Table 3-2 Troubleshooting hemodynamic monitoring systems

Problem	Cause	Corrective Action
No waveform	No power supply, loose connection	Turn on power, check all connections
	Stopcocks are turned off to patient	Properly position stopcocks
	Catheter is occluded or has moved out of the vessel	Attempt to aspirate clot, reposition the catheter*
Artifact	Electrical interference	Have electrical equipment in room checked
	Patient movement	Request the patient to lie quietly
	Catheter whip	Reposition catheter;* monitor on "mean," try longer/shorter monitoring tubing
Drifting waveform	Temperature change of IV flush solution	Allow temperature of solution to stabilize
	Monitor cable is kinked or compressed	Check cable and relieve kink or compression
Unable to flush line	Stopcock turned off	Properly position stopcock
	Tubing kinked	Relieve kink in tubing
	Pressure bag not adequately inflated	Inflate pressure bag to 300 mm Hg
False high reading	Improper calibration	Recalibrate
	Transducer below the phlebostatic axis	Reposition transducer
	Catheter kinked	Reposition catheter*
	Catheter tip occluded	Attempt to aspirate clot
	Catheter tip resting against vessel wall	Reposition catheter*

Problem		Cause	Intervention
False low reading		Improper calibration	Recalibrate
		Transducer above the phlebostatic axis	Reposition transducer
		Loose connection	Tighten all connections
		Air bubbles in system	Aspirate all air from system
Dampened waveform		Tubing kinked	Check for kinks in tubing
		Loose connection	Tighten all connections
		Catheter tip occluded	Attempt to aspirate clot
		Catheter tip resting against vessel wall	Reposition catheter*
		Pressure bag not adequately inflated	Inflate pressure bag to 300 mm Hg
Inability to wedge		Balloon rupture	Do not continue to inject air into balloon, replace with properly functioning catheter
Overwedging		Improper catheter position	Reposition catheter*
		Catheter migration into PA	Reposition catheter*
Spontaneous wedging		Catheter migration into wedge position without inflation of balloon	Reposition catheter*
Ventricular dysrhythmias		Catheter migration into RV	Reposition catheter*

*Temporary repositioning of the catheter may be achieved by having the patient turn to the right or left or by having the patient cough. Generally only the physician should manually manipulate the catheter. Waveforms from Daily E, Schroeder J: *Hemodynamic waveforms*, St Louis, 1993, Mosby.

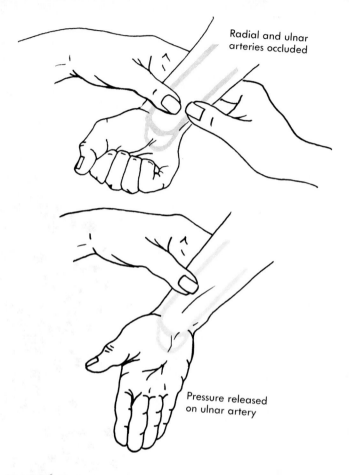

Figure 3-6
Allen test. Hold patient's hand up. Ask patient to clench and unclench hand while you occlude the radial and ulnar arteries. The hand will become pale. Lower the hand and have the patient relax the hand. While continuing to occlude the radial artery, release pressure on the ulnar artery. A brisk return of color in a period of 5 to 7 seconds demonstrates adequate ulnar blood flow. If pallor persists for more than 15 seconds, ulnar flow is inadequate and radial artery cannulation should not be attempted.

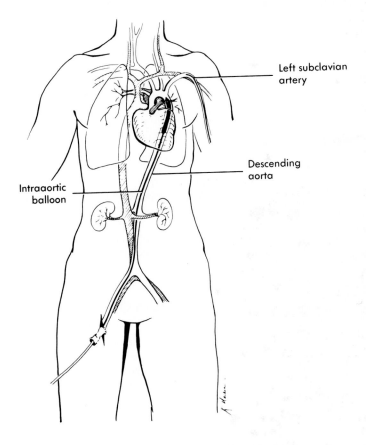

Left subclavian
artery

Descending
aorta

Intraaortic
balloon

Figure 3-7
**Intra-aortic balloon pump position. The balloon is positioned
in the descending thoracic aorta.**
From Quaal S: *Comprehensive intra-aortic balloon counterpulsation,* St Louis, 1993,
Mosby.

Indications

- Cardiogenic shock
- Severe left ventricular failure
- Severe unstable angina
- Postinfarction angina
- Refractory ventricular dysrhythmias
- Decreased tissue perfusion

Hemodynamic effects

Increased supply
- ↑ diastolic aortic pressure
- ↑ coronary perfusion
- ↑ cerebral and renal perfusion
- ↑ stroke volume, ejection fraction, cardiac output

Decreased demand
- ↓ myocardial oxygen consumption
- ↓ afterload (systolic pressure, systemic vascular resistance)
- ↓ preload (left ventricular diastolic pressure, left atrial pressure, pulmonary artery wedge pressure)
- ↓ heart rate

Timing of balloon inflation and deflation

Ideal timing maximizes the hemodynamic effects achieved with the IABP. Balloon inflation should begin at the dicrotic notch (aortic valve closure), with balloon deflation occurring just before the aortic valve opens. Triggering of inflation and deflation is generally done from the ECG (Figure 3-8); timing is adjusted from the arterial waveform (Figure 3-9). Timing is evaluated with the balloon on a 1:2 assist mode (balloon inflates every other beat). When timing is ideal, balloon-assisted end diastolic pressure will be 5 to 15 mm Hg lower than the patient's (unassisted) diastolic pressure. Balloon-assisted systolic pressure will be lower than the patient's (unassisted) systolic pressure. Because of the lower assisted end diastolic pressure, less pressure is required for systole following balloon inflation and thus, work for the ventricle is decreased.

Discontinuation of the IABP

Weaning from the IABP is done over the course of several hours. The following criteria are used:

1. Hemodynamic stability with minimal vasopressor support
   - Cardiac index > 2 L/min/m^2

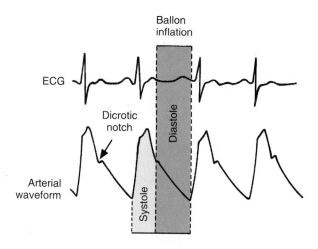

Figure 3-8
IABP—period of balloon inflation.

Figure 3-9
Arterial waveform with balloon inflating every other beat. *1,*
Balloon-assisted aortic end diastolic pressure; *2,* patient aortic
end diastolic pressure; *3,* balloon-assisted systole; *4,* patient
systole; *5,* peak diastolic augmented pressure.
From Quaal S: *Comprehensive intra-aortic balloon counterpulsation,* St Louis,
1993, Mosby.

- PAWP ≤ 18-20 mm Hg
- Systolic BP > 100 mm Hg
2. Adequate cardiac function
  - Urine output > 30 ml/hour
  - Improved mentation
  - No crackles, no S_3

3. Adequate coronary perfusion
   · No life-threatening dysrhythmias
   · No ischemia on ECG
   · Heart rate < 110 beats/minute

Discontinuation of the IABP without weaning may be necessary for the following reasons: severe vascular insufficiency, indicated by loss of pulse and cold, cyanotic extremities; balloon leakage; deterioration of an irreversible condition; or inability to wean.

Troubleshooting

Common problems encountered with use of the IABP, along with cause and corrective action, can be found in Table 3-3.

Clinical Alert

Monitor hemodynamic and clinical status on a continuous basis.
Assess circulation (pulses, temperature, and color) to extremities (especially distal to balloon insertion site and left arm) every 1 to 2 hours. If the balloon migrates upward, flow through the left subclavian will be impeded, decreasing perfusion to the left arm.
Immobilize leg in which the balloon is inserted.
Raise head of bed to an angle no higher than 30°.
Change dressing over insertion site every 24 to 48 hours, or according to hospital policy.
A balloon left deflated for more than 5 minutes predisposes the patient to thrombus formation—manually inflate if necessary.
If the patient is receiving anticoagulants, monitor appropriate coagulation studies and observe for bleeding.

Pacemakers

Description

A pacemaker is a device that provides electrical impulses that restore regular rhythm or increase heart rate to achieve improved cardiac output and tissue perfusion. A temporary pacemaker is equipped with an external pulse generator. A permanent pacemaker contains an implanted pulse generator. Pacing can be done via endocardial electrodes (placed transvenously), epicardial electrodes (placed via thoracotomy), or chest wall electrodes (placed transcutaneously). Pacemakers can be programmed to function only when needed (demand) or to function regardless of the patient's intrinsic rhythm (fixed rate).

✳ Table 3-3 Troubleshooting the intra-aortic balloon pump

Problem	Cause	Corrective Action
Loss of dicrotic notch	Early balloon inflation	Change timing to delay balloon inflation
Balloon inflation after dicrotic notch	Late balloon inflation	Change timing so balloon inflates at the dicrotic notch
Rise in assisted systolic pressure	Early balloon deflation	Change timing to delay balloon deflation
Rise in assisted diastolic pressure	Late balloon deflation	Change timing so balloon deflates before the next systole
Alarm for impaired gas movement goes off	Kink in catheter	Straighten catheter, if kinked
Low gas alarm goes off	Leak in balloon, rupture of balloon	Refill balloon q 2-4 hours (if manual system); assess patient for gas embolism; assist with removal of balloon and replacement if necessary
Inadequate balloon inflation/deflation	Arterial monitoring system not calibrated	Calibrate system
	Poor arterial tracing	Remove any air from system; flush system; if catheter occluded, attempt to aspirate clot
	Poor ECG tracing	Replace any loose electrodes; place electrodes to maximize R wave height

Indications

- Bradydysrhythmias
- Heart blocks
- Recurrent ventricular tachycardia
- Sick sinus syndrome
- Tachydysrhythmias unresponsive to drugs (overdrive pacing)

Classification

The Inter-Society Commission for Heart Disease Resources (ICHD) pacemaker code, consisting of three letters, was developed in 1974. Several revisions have been made to this code as a result of advancements in pacemaker technology. The most recent revision, made in 1987 by the North American Society of Pacing and Electrophysiology (NASPE) and the British Pacing and Electrophysiology Group (BPEG), consists of five letters and is referred to as the NBG (NASPE/BPEG generic) pacemaker code (Table 3-4). The first three letters of the NBG Code are the same as the original ICHD code. Application of the code to identify pacemakers can be found in Table 3-5.

Pacemaker malfunction

Most pacemaker malfunctions are caused by failure to sense, to capture, or to pace. Common causes for these malfunctions, as well as corrective actions, are found in Table 3-6.

Clinical Alert

- Assess for proper pacing, capture, and sensing.
- Monitor patient's hemodynamic and clinical status.
- Change dressing per hospital policy or physician's orders.
- Temporary pacemakers: wear rubber gloves when handling generator or leads, place exposed wires in rubber glove, do not handle other electrical equipment while holding generator or leads, be sure all electrical equipment is grounded, do not allow patient to use electrical equipment.

Implantable Cardioverter Defibrillator (ICD)

Description

The ICD consists of a pulse generator and two lead (sensing) systems that continuously monitor heart activity and automatically deliver a low-energy shock when ventricular tachydysrhythmias are detected. Battery life expectancy is 3 to 4 years or 300 30-joule shocks.

Table 3-4   **NBG pacemaker code**

I. Chamber(s) paced	O-None
	A-Atrium
	V-Ventricle
	D-Dual (atrium and ventricle)
II. Chamber(s) sensed	O-None
	A-Atrium
	V-Ventricle
	D-Dual (atrium and ventricle)
III. Response to sensing	O-None
	T-Triggered
	I-Inhibited
	D-Dual (triggered and inhibited)
IV. Programmability, rate modulation	O-None
	P-Simple programmable
	M-Multiprogrammable
	C-Communicating
	R-Rate modulation
V. Antitachyarrhythmia function(s)	O-None
	P-Pacing (antitachyarrhythmia)
	S-Shock
	D-Dual (pacing and shock)

From Bernstein A: *Pace* 10:795, 1987.

Table 3-5   **Examples of pacemakers using the NBG code**

AAIOO	Atrial pacing, atrial sensing, a sensed atrial event inhibits pacing, no programmability, no antitachyarrhythmia function
VVIRO	Ventricular pacing, ventricular sensing, a sensed ventricular event inhibits pacing, adaptive rate response, no antitachyarrhythmia function
DVICO	Atrial and ventricular pacing, ventricular sensing, inhibited atrial and ventricular response to ventricular sensing, multiprogrammable with telemetry, no antitachyarrhythmia function
DDDCO	Atrial and ventricular pacing, atrial and ventricular sensing, inhibited atrial and ventricular response to atrial and ventricular sensing, triggered ventricular response to atrial sensing, multiprogrammable with telemetry, no antitachyarrhythmia function

Table 3-6 Pacemaker malfunction

Problem	Cause	Corrective Action
Failure to sense	Displaced lead, fixed rate pacing	Turn patient to left side, increase sensitivity of generator, turn pacer off if not needed (leave in place should pacing be required)
Failure to capture	Inadequate electrical output, displaced lead	Increase pacer output (MA), turn patient on left side, reposition lead
Failure to pace (no pacer spikes)	Generator or battery failure, loose connection between lead and generator, inhibition of generator due to interference by extraneous signal	Check on/off setting, replace generator or battery, check connections, reprogram
	Fractured lead	Replace lead

Rhythm strips from Conover M: *Pocket nurse guide to electrocardiography*, St Louis, 1990, Mosby.

Indications

- Survival from near sudden death caused by unstable tachydysrhythmias not associated with acute myocardial infarction
- Recurrent refractory life-threatening ventricular dysrhythmias, despite conventional antidysrhythmic drug therapy

Contraindications

- Concomitant disease with less than 1 year expected survival
- Incidence of nonsustained ventricular tachycardia
- Multiple daily episodes of life-threatening dysrhythmias

Malfunction

- Repeated, inappropriate, false-positive shocks indicate malfunction. Notify the physician, who will determine whether to inactivate the device. Electromagnetic interference (i.e., diathermy or magnetic resonance imagers) may cause either inhibition of sensing or inappropriate discharge.

Clinical Alert

- Note if the ICD is in the active or inactive mode. Some physicians elect to leave the ICD in the inactive mode for several days. In the early postoperative period, transient episodes of supraventricular or nonsustained ventricular tachycardia are not uncommon.
- If the ICD is in the inactive mode and symptomatic sustained VT/VF occurs, institute routine emergency procedures (CPR or countershock). Cardioversion or defibrillation can be performed externally without damage to the ICD.
- If the ICD is in the active mode, electrical shock will be given 10 to 35 seconds after dysrhythmia is sensed. If dysrhythmia is not terminated by the first shock, the ICD will recharge and deliver three more shocks. The ICD will not recycle until 35 seconds of nonshockable rhythm (asystole, heart block, junctional or sinus rhythm) is detected by the sensors. If VT/VF remains after the four shocks, institute routine emergency procedures. Some ICD's will give a total of five shocks.
- Anyone touching the patient at the time of ICD discharge may experience up to a 2-joule shock.

Cardioverter/Defibrillator

Description

Cardioversion and defibrillation are procedures that use electric current to terminate select cardiac dysrhythmias. The electrical current causes depolarization of myocardial cells, disrupting the dysrhythmia. Cardioversion differs from defibrillation in that the defibrillator is synchronized to deliver the electrical current approximately 10 msec after the peak of the R wave. This is to avoid accidental delivery of the current during the T wave, which may result in ventricular fibrillation.

Clinical Alert

- Place one paddle at the second intercostal space right of the sternum and the second paddle at the left precordium (fifth intercostal space, anterior axillary line). Confirm dysrhythmia. Exert 25 pounds paddle pressure during delivery of current.
- Do not place paddles over nitroglycerin ointment or transdermal patch.
- Avoid smearing conductive gel over the patient's chest or on paddle handles or placing paddles over ECG monitoring electrodes or permanent pulse generator (paddles should be at least 5 inches from generator).
- Before discharging paddles, disconnect temporary pacemaker or other electrical equipment. Be sure that personnel are clear of bed, patient, and equipment.
- Defibrillation may also be accomplished via an automated external defibrillator (AED), a device that incorporates an external defibrillator with a cardiac rhythm analysis system. The device has two adhesive pads applied to the patient's chest that will sense and record the cardiac rhythm and, if necessary, deliver an electrical shock.

Selected bibliography

Alspach J editor: *Core curriculum for critical care nursing,* Philadelphia, 1991, Saunders.

Bernstein A and others: The NASPE/BPEG generic pacemaker code for antibradyarrhythmia and adaptive-rate pacing and antitachyarrhythmia devices, *PACE* 10:794-799, 1987.

Boggs R, Wooldridge-King M, editors: *Procedure manual for critical care,* Philadelphia, 1993, Saunders.

Daily E, Schroeder J: *Hemodynamic waveforms,* St Louis, 1993, Mosby.

Darovic G: *Hemodynamic monitoring,* Philadelphia, 1987, Saunders.

Jafri S, Kruse J: Temporary transvenous cardiac pacing, *Critical Care Clinics* 8(4):713-726, 1992.

Lehmann M, Saksena S: Implantable cardioverter defibrillators in cardiovascular practice: report of the policy conference of the North American Society of Pacing and Electrophysiology, *PACE* 14(6):969-979, 1991.

Martin M, Aragon D: Temporary DDD pacing: evaluating hemodynamic performance, *Dimensions of Critical Care* 11(4):191-200, 1992.

Mason P. McPherson C: Implantable cardioverter defibrillator: a review, *Heart Lung* 21(2):141-147, 1992.

Noone J: Troubleshooting pulmonary artery catheters, *Critical Care Nurse* 8(2):52-64, 1988.

Quaal S: *Comprehensive intra-aortic balloon counterpulsation,* St Louis, 1993, Mosby.

Schermer L: Physiologic and technical variables affecting hemodynamic measurements, *Critical Care Nurse* 8(2):33-42, 1988.

Swearingen P, Keen J, editors: *Manual of critical care,* St Louis, 1991, Mosby.

Textbook of advanced cardiac life support, Dallas, 1990, American Heart Association.

Cardiovascular Pharmacologic Agents

4

The following groups of drugs are discussed in this chapter: sympathomimetic, sympatholytic, parasympatholytic, antianginal, antidysrhythmic, cardiotonic, diuretic, antihypertensive, antihyperlipidemic, and hematologic agents, as well as drugs used to treat peripheral vascular disease.

These drugs, when used alone or in combination, can have beneficial effects on cardiac output and blood vessel patency. However, a patient's hemodynamic status must be carefully monitored because serious adverse effects may also occur. Multiple drug therapy can produce additive or potentiated drug effects. In addition, when a drug is added or removed from a patient's regimen, the patient's response to therapy must be critically evaluated because drug blood concentrations may be altered. Drug serum levels can be used to determine if the concentration level of the drug is between the minimum effective concentration and the minimum toxic concentration (that is, within the therapeutic range). However, patients may experience signs and symptoms of toxicity yet exhibit drug blood concentrations within the established acceptable therapeutic range. Any condition that alters the pharmacokinetics (absorption, distribution, metabolism, and excretion) of a drug, such as impaired hepatic or renal function, can increase a patient's risk for toxic drug effects. Therefore evaluation of renal and liver function tests and close clinical observation of the patient for the onset of adverse effects are critical.

Autonomic Nervous System

Overview

The cardiovascular system is regulated by the two divisions of the autonomic nervous system, the sympathetic and parasympathetic systems. These two divisions provide a physiologically balanced internal environment.

Sympathetic nervous system (SNS) stimulation results in a response referred to as the "adrenergic response" because of the release of the neurotransmitter norepinephrine (adrenalin). Neurotransmitters for the SNS are commonly referred to as catecholamines and include epinephrine and dopamine in addition to norepinephrine. A "cholinergic" or "vagal" response describes the response to parasympathetic nervous system (PNS) stimulation. The neurotransmitter for the PNS is acetylcholine (See Table 4-1 for a comparison of responses of the SNS and PNS.)

Both inhibitory and excitatory responses can result from stimulation of the SNS. This is due in part to two different adrenergic receptor types. These receptors, referred to as alpha and beta receptors, are subdivided into alpha 1, alpha 2, beta 1, and beta 2. Alpha receptors are located in vascular smooth muscle. Beta 1 receptors are located in the heart, beta 2 receptors are located in vascular smooth muscle and bronchi.

Dopaminergic receptors are found in coronary, renal, and mesenteric blood vessels. Stimulation of these receptors results in coronary, renal, and mesenteric artery dilatation. A summary of receptor responses can be found in the box below. Stimulation of the autonomic nervous system also produces noncardiac effects. (See Table 4-1).

✕ Receptor Responses

Receptor	Response
Beta 1	↑ HR, ↑ myocardial contractility resulting in ↑ SV and ↑ CO, ↑ myocardial oxygen consumption
Beta 2	↑ Coronary blood flow, vasodilatation of bronchial smooth muscle
Alpha	Vasoconstriction resulting in ↑ SBP and ↑ DBP, ↑ peripheral vascular resistance
Dopaminergic	Renal, mesenteric, and cerebral vasodilatation; renal vasodilatation causes ↑ renal blood flow, resulting in increase glomerular filtration and ↑ urine output

---

CO, cardiac output; DBP, diastolic blood pressure; HR, heart rate; SBP, systolic blood pressure; SV, stroke volume.

Table 4-1   Responses to autonomic nervous system
stimulation

	Sympathetic Stimulation	Parasympathetic Stimulation
Cardiac Effects		
Rate of impulse formation	Increased	Decreased
Force of contraction	Increased	Decreased
Speed of impulse conduction	Increased	Decreased
Myocardial oxygen demand	Increased	Decreased
Coronary arteries	Dilatation (beta 2); constriction (alpha)	Dilatation
Vascular Effects		
Arteries and arterioles	Constriction (alpha); dilatation (dopaminergic)	None
Veins	Constriction	None
Major Systemic Effects		
Eye	Pupillary dilatation	Pupillary constriction
Bronchi	Dilatation	Constriction
Gut	Decreased peristalsis	Increased peristalsis
Liver	Increased glycogenolysis	None
Kidney	Decreased urine output; increased renin secretion	None

Continuous exposure to catecholamines may reduce the number of adrenergic receptors (known as "down regulation") and the affinity of these receptors for sympathomimetic drugs. A decrease in the responsiveness (refractoriness, desensitization, tachyphylaxis) of the end organ may result. Since sympathetic nervous system activity is increased with conditions such as congestive heart failure, patients may become refractory to sympathomimetic agents, requiring increased dosages or a change in drug therapy. "Up regulation" (an increase in receptor number) may occur in patients receiving adrenergic blocking agents, causing a hyperadrenergic state when the agent is withdrawn. This phenomenon may explain the signs and symptoms associated with abrupt withdrawal of propranolol (Inderal). Dosage should be gradually reduced when discontinuing such agents.

A variety of terms has been used to classify pharmacologic agents that produce sympathetic and parasympathetic nervous system responses. Drugs that mimic the sympathetic response are referred to as sympathomimetics, adrenergic stimulating agents, or adrenergic agonists. Drugs that block the sympathetic response are referred to as sympatholytics, adrenergic blockers, or adrenergic antagonists. Drugs that initiate the parasympathetic response are referred to as parasympathomimetics, cholinergic stimulating agents, or cholinergic agonists. Drugs that block the parasympathetic response are referred to as parasympatholytics, cholinergic blockers, cholinergic antagonists, or anticholinergic agents.

Sympathomimetic Agents

The adrenergic stimulating agents are summarized in Table 4-2.

Table 4-2   **Adrenergic stimulating agents**

Drug and Receptor	Indication and Usual Dosage
Dobutamine (Dobutrex)— *beta 1, beta 2*	Congestive heart failure or cardiogenic shock: Infusion 500 mg/250 ml D$_5$W (1 ml = 2000 µg); at 2.0-20 µg/kg/min
Dopamine (Intropin)— *dopaminergic, beta 1, alpha*	Hypotension or cardiogenic shock: Infusion 800 mg/500 ml D$_5$W (1 ml = 1600 µg); low dose = 1-2 µg/kg/min; moderate dose = 2-10 µg/kg/min; high dose >10 µg/kg/min

Continued.

Table 4-2   Adrenergic stimulating agents—cont'd

Drug and Receptor	Indication and Usual Dosage	
Epinephrine (Adrenalin)— *beta 1, beta 2, alpha*	Anaphylaxis:	
	SQ or IM	0.1-0.5 ml of 1:1000 solution
	IV	0.1-0.25 ml of 1:1000 solution
	Hypotension:	
	Infusion	1 mg/500 ml D_5W; 1 µg/min, titrate to desired effect
	Cardiac arrest:	
	IV	1 mg of 1:10,000 solution; repeat q3-5 minutes
	Endotracheal	Optimal dose is unknown, may need 2-2.5 times peripheral IV dose; follow with 5-10 forceful inhalations
	Infusion	30 mg/250 ml D_5W; titrate to desired effect (i.e., blood pressure, cardiac output)
Isoproterenol (Isuprel)— *beta 1, beta 2*	Hemodynamic significant bradycardia or refractory torsades de pointes:	
	Infusion	1 mg/500 ml D_5W (1 ml = 2 µg); at 2-10 µg/min; titrate to pulse of 60
Metaraminol (Aramine)— *beta 1, alpha*	Cardiogenic shock or hypotension:	
	IV	0.5-5 mg followed by:
	Infusion	100 mg/250 ml D_5W (1 ml = 400 µg); titrate to desired blood pressure
Norepinephrine (Levophed)— *beta 1, alpha*	Hypotension:	
	Infusion	4 mg/250 ml D_5W (1 ml = 16 µg); titrate to desired blood pressure

Adrenergic Stimulating Agents

Description

Adrenergic stimulating agents mimic the responses of the sympathetic nervous system to produce peripheral vasoconstriction, cardiac stimulation, bronchial relaxation, and vasodilation of vessels supplying the heart, brain, kidneys, and skeletal muscle. Although the increase in blood pressure, heart rate, contractility, and bronchiole diameter are desirable effects in select cardiovascular problems, the simultaneous increase in myocardial oxygen consumption is not. These agents are used to treat hypotension, shock, congestive heart failure, and cardiac arrest. Major cardiovascular side effects include hypertension, chest pain, palpitations, and dysrhythmias.

Clinical Alert

Concurrent use of adrenergic stimulating agents and other drugs that affect cardiovascular function may potentiate or antagonize the pharmacologic effects of these agents.

Administration Precautions: Adrenergic Stimulating Agents

- Do not administer these drugs via the proximal port of a pulmonary artery catheter if thermodilution cardiac outputs are being obtained.
- Intravenous infusions should be administered by an IV infusion device to control the amount of drug delivered to the patient.
- Intra-arterial pressure monitoring is recommended during administration of these agents.
- Check proper functioning of equipment, validate correct drug concentration and infusion rate.
- Use large veins whenever possible. Check IV site frequently; if blanching, a preliminary sign of extravasation, occurs along the vein, change IV site. If extravasation occurs, use a large-gauge needle to infiltrate the area liberally with phentolamine (Regitine), 5-10 mg in 10-15 ml of normal saline.
- Exercise caution in patients with peripheral vascular occlusive disease; drugs with alpha properties can cause excessive vasoconstriction.

Patient Assessment: Adrenergic Stimulating Agents

- Blood pressure and heart rate should be checked every 2-5 minutes during initiation and titration of these drugs.

- Closely evaluate pulse pressure and other hemodynamic parameters of cardiac output (see Appendix C).
- Check IV site frequently.

Patient Adverse Effects: Adrenergic Stimulating Agents

- Signs of excessive alpha effects: numbness, tingling, pallor, cold skin temperature, diminished or absent pulses, decreased urine output, and decreased cerebral perfusion.
- Chest pain, tachycardia, dysrhythmias, headache, restlessness, hypertension, hypotension, shortness of breath, and pulmonary edema.
- Unresponsiveness to increasing doses of the drug.

Administration Precautions: Specific Agents

Dobutamine

- Do not administer to patients with hypertrophic cardiomyopathy; outflow tract gradient may worsen.
- A rapid ventricular response may result if dobutamine is administered to a patient in atrial fibrillation. The patient should receive a digitalis preparation.

Dopamine

- Do not administer to patients with pheochromocytoma; severe hypertension may result.
- Effects of morphine are antagonized; patients may need increased dosages of the analgesic.
- Hypovolemia should be corrected before this drug is used for its vasopressor effects.

Epinephrine

- Do not administer concurrently with isoproterenol (Isuprel); death may result.
- Hypovolemia should be corrected before this drug is used for its vasopressor effects.
- Do not use to treat an overdose of adrenergic blocking agents, since irreversible shock may occur.
- Hyperglycemia may develop.

Isoproterenol

- Isoproterenol is not indicated in cardiac arrest.
- Do not use concurrently with epinephrine; death may result.

- Serious dysrhythmias can develop; isoproterenol may cause ventricular fibrillation and ventricular tachycardia.

Metaraminol

- Hypovolemia should be corrected before this drug is used for its vasopressor effects.
- Pulmonary edema may result from a rapid rise in blood pressure.

Norepinephrine

- Hypovolemia should be corrected before this drug is used for its vasopressor effects.
- Volume depletion and a decrease in cardiac output secondary to increased peripheral vascular resistance may occur with prolonged use.
- Hyperglycemia may develop.

Sympatholytic Agents

Beta adrenergic blocking agents are summarized in Table 4-3. Alpha adrenergic blocking agents are discussed on p. 204.

Table 4-3   **Beta adrenergic blocking agents**

Drug and Selectivity	Indication and Usual Dosage	
Acebutolol (Sectral) *ISA, beta 1*	Dysrhythmias:	
	Oral	200 mg q12hr
	Range	600-1200 mg qd
	High blood pressure:	
	Oral	400 mg qd
	Range	200-1200 mg qd
Atenolol (Tenormin) *beta 1*	Angina and high blood pressure:	
	Oral	25-50 mg qd
	Range	50-100 mg qd
	Myocardial reinfarction prophylaxis:	
	IV	5 mg, repeat in 10 minutes; then
	Oral	50 mg 10 min after last IV dose, 50 mg 12 hrs later, 100 mg qd

Continued.

Table 4-3 Beta adrenergic blocking agents—cont'd

Drug and Selectivity	Indication and Usual Dosage	
Betaxolol (Kerlone) *beta 1*	High blood pressure:	
	Oral	10 mg qd
Carteolol (Cartrol) *ISA, nonselective*	Angina and high blood pressure:	
	Oral	2.5-5.0 mg qd
	Maxi- mum	10 mg qd
Esmolol (Brevibloc) *beta 1*	Supraventricular tachycardia:	
	Infusion	5 g/500 ml D_5W (1 ml = 10 mg); loading dose: 500 µg/kg/min—for 1 minute; then 50 µg/kg/min for 4 minutes. If desired response is not achieved, repeat the loading dose, then, infuse 100 µg/kg/min for 4 minutes. Continue to repeat loading dose and increase maintenance dose in increments of 50 µg/kg/min until the desired rhythm is achieved.
	Maxi- mum	200 µg/kg/min
Labetalol (Trandate, Normodyne) *nonselective, beta 1, beta 2, alpha*	High blood pressure:	
	Oral	100 mg bid
	Range	200-400 mg bid
	IV	20 mg over 2 minutes; additional injections of 40 mg and 80 mg may be given every 10 minutes up to 300 mg; or:
	Infusion	200 mg/160 ml D_5W (1 ml = 1 mg); 2 mg/min; titrate to desired blood pressure

ISA, Intrinsic sympathetic activity.

Table 4-3   Beta adrenergic blocking agents—cont'd

Drug and Selectivity	Indication and Usual Dosage	
Metoprolol (Lopressor) *beta 1*	Angina or high blood pressure:	
	Oral	100 mg qd
	Range	100-450 mg qd
	Myocardial reinfarction prophylaxis:	
	IV	5 mg ×3 doses, 2 minutes apart; wait 15 minutes then:
	Oral	50 mg q6h ×48h; then 100 mg q 12h
Nadolol (Corgard) *nonselective*	Angina:	
	Oral	40 mg qd
	Range	80-240 mg qd
	High blood pressure:	
	Oral	40 mg qd
	Maximum	320 mg qd
Penbutolol (Levatol) *ISA, nonselective*	Angina or high blood pressure:	
	Oral	20 mg qd
	Range	20-80 mg qd
Pindolol (Visken) *ISA, nonselective*	High blood pressure:	
	Oral	5 mg bid
	Maximum	60 mg qd
Propranolol (Inderal) *nonselective*	High blood pressure:	
	Oral	40 mg bid
	Maximum	640 mg qd
	Sustained release capsules	80-160 mg qd
	Angina:	
	Oral	10-20 mg tid-qid
	Maximum	320 mg qd
	Dysrhythmias:	
	Oral	10-30 mg tid-qid
	IV	1-3 mg (1 mg/min); wait 2-3 minutes; repeat if necessary
	Myocardial reinfarction prophylaxis:	
	Oral	180-240 mg qd in divided doses

Continued.

Table 4-3   Beta adrenergic blocking agents—cont'd

Drug and Selectivity	Indication and Usual Dosage	
Propranolol—cont'd	Obstructive hypertrophic cardiomyopathy:	
	Oral	20-40 mg tid-qid
	Sustained-release capsules	80-160 mg qd
Timolol (Blocadren) *nonselective*	High blood pressure:	
	Oral	10 mg bid
	Range	20-80 mg qd
	Myocardial reinfarction prophylaxis:	
	Oral	10 mg bid initiated 1-4 weeks post-MI

Beta Adrenergic Blocking Agents

Description

Beta adrenergic blocking agents block beta receptor sites. The adrenergic response is thus blocked, resulting in decreased heart rate, contractility, and blood pressure. Reducing afterload and heart rate decreases myocardial oxygen demand. The reduction in heart rate allows for a longer diastolic filling time, which improves coronary perfusion. Beta adrenergic blocking effects improve exercise tolerance in patients with angina.

Some beta blocking agents possess a cardioselective property—that is, they have a preference for blocking beta 1 receptors (see Table 4-3). These agents produce limited adverse effects on the pulmonary system, unlike nonselective beta blockers, which affect both beta 1 and beta 2 receptors and are therefore capable of producing bronchospasm. As dosage needs increase, however, cardioselective agents begin to block beta 2 receptors as well as beta 1 receptors.

Some beta blockers exhibit intrinsic sympathetic activity (ISA), causing a weak stimulation of beta adrenergic receptors. These drugs cause little slowing of heart rate and are useful in patients who are bradycardic and have minimal cardiac reserve (See Table 4-3). Because of the effects on the cardiovascular system, beta blockers are used to treat a variety of cardiovascular conditions, in cluding angina pectoris, high blood pressure, supraventricular and ventricular dysrhythmias, mitral valve prolapse, and obstructive hypertrophic cardiomyopathy. Major cardiovascular side effects include orthostatic hypotension, bradycardia and other dysrhythmias, heart failure, and aggravation of peripheral vascular disease.

Clinical Alert

Concurrent use of beta adrenergic blocking agents and other drugs that affect cardiovascular function may potentiate or antagonize the pharmacologic effects of the drugs.

Administration Precautions: Beta Adrenergic Blocking Agents

- Do not administer to patients with bradycardia (<45 bpm), heart block, hypotension (SBP < 90 mm Hg), or overt cardiac failure. Check heart rate and blood pressure before drug administration.
- Be prepared to administer atropine if severe bradycardia occurs.
- Glucagon may be given to reverse the cardiovascular effects of bradycardia and hypotension.
- Do not administer nonselective beta blockers to patients with asthma.
- Diabetic patients may develop hyperglycemia or hypoglycemia as a result of the drug's blocking effect on insulin release and its masking of signs and symptoms of hypoglycemia.
- Reduced dosages may be required in patients with impaired renal or hepatic function.
- Angina, dysrhythmias, or myocardial infarction may result if beta blocking agents are abruptly withdrawn.

Patient Assessment: Beta Adrenergic Blocking Agents

- Assess if the dysrhythmia is resolved, anginal episodes are reduced, or hypertension is controlled.
- See Reportable Adverse Effects, which follow.

Reportable Adverse Effects: Beta Adrenergic Blocking Agents

- Systolic blood pressure <90 mm Hg, heart rate <50 bpm, or development of dizziness or decreased level of consciousness.

- Signs and symptoms of heart failure: crackles, S_3, shortness of breath, or ankle edema.
- Development of wheezing and difficulty with breathing.
- Altered glucose levels, signs and symptoms of hypoglycemia or hyperglycemia.
- Withdrawal signs: chest pain, tachycardia, irregular rhythm, sudden shortness of breath, sweating, or trembling.
- Signs and symptoms of overdosage: tachycardia, bradycardia, a change in heart rhythm, dizziness or fainting, difficulty breathing, bluish-colored fingernails or palmar surface of the hands, or seizures. Other indications include cold hands or feet, back or joint pain, confusion, mental depression, fever, sore throat, and unusual bleeding.

Parasympatholytic Agent

The cholinergic blocking agent (anticholinergic agent) is summarized in Table 4-4.

Cholinergic Blocking Agent

Description

Atropine produces an increase in heart rate and contractility. These effects result from the blocking action of acetylcholine, leaving the sympathetic nervous system unopposed. Atropine is used to treat symptomatic bradycardia and asystole. Major cardiovascular side effects include tachycardia and increased ischemia and extension of infarction zones in MI patients.

Administration Precautions: Atropine

- Atropine is indicated in patients with symptomatic bradycardia: associated hypotension, ventricular ectopy, or myocardial ischemia.
- Administering less than 0.5 mg has parasympathomimetic effects and can produce paradoxic bradycardia. Ventricular fibrillation can develop as a result of this effect.
- Myocardial oxygen demand is increased as a result of increased heart rate. Use cautiously in patients with MI or angina.
- Atropine is contraindicated in acute glaucoma, myasthenia gravis, and obstructive GI and GU conditions.

Table 4-4   Cholinergic blocking agent (anticholinergic)

Drug	Indication and Usual Dosage	
Atropine	Bradycardia:	
	IV	0.5-1.0 mg q 3-5 min until desired response is achieved (heart rate >60 bpm); or up to 0.04 mg/kg
	Asystole:	
	IV	1 mg; repeat q 3-5 min up to a total of 0.04 mg/kg
	Endotracheal	2-2.5 times the recommended IV dose may be diluted in 10 ml normal saline; follow with 5 forceful inhalations

Patient Assessment: Atropine

· Monitor heart rate; a rate >60 bpm is desirable.
· See Reportable Adverse Effects, which follow.

Reportable Adverse Effects: Atropine

· Excessive doses can produce tachycardia, flushed hot skin, delirium, coma, or death.

Antianginal Agents

Overview

Antianginal agents decrease myocardial oxygen demand and improve coronary artery blood flow. See Table 1-1 for factors that determine myocardial oxygen supply and demand. Pharmacologic agents that manipulate oxygen supply and demand are used to treat angina and include nitrates, calcium channel blockers, and beta adrenergic blockers.

Nitrates are the most frequently used antianginal agent and can be used in combination with beta adrenergic blocking agents and/or calcium channel blocking agents. Beta adrenergic blocking agents have been found to prevent reinfarction after MI; therefore, they are frequently used to treat patients with stable angina who have had a MI. Calcium channel blocking agents are effective in preventing coronary artery spasm of variant angina and may also be the drug of choice to control angina in patients with diabetes or vascular disease. A summary of antianginal agents can be found in Table 4-5.

Nitrates

Table 4-6 summarizes the nitrates with indications and dosages.

Table 4-5 **Antianginal agents and effects on oxygen supply and demand**

	Nitrates	Beta Blockers	Calcium Channel Blockers
Oxygen Demand Determinants			
Heart rate	↑	↓	↓*
Contractility	—	↓	↓
Preload	↓	—	—
Afterload	↓	↓	↓
Oxygen Supply Determinants			
Coronary artery diameter	↑	—	↑
Diastolic filling time	—**	↑	↑

*Nifedipine and nicardipine may cause reflex tachycardia.
**May decrease as a result of reflex tachycardia.
—No effect.

Table 4-6 **Nitrates**

Drug	Indication and Usual Dosage	
Isosorbide dinitrate (Isordil)	Prophylaxis:	
	Sublingual	2.5-10 mg q 2-3h
	Oral	5-20 mg q 6h
	Range	5-40 mg 4×/day
	Sustained release	40-80 mg q 8-12h
	Chewable	5-10 mg q 2-3h
Isosorbide mononitrate (ISMO)	Prophylaxis:	
	Oral	20 mg bid

Table 4-6 **Nitrates**—cont'd

Drug	Indication and Usual Dosage	
Nitroglycerin (Nitrostat)	Acute attacks: Sublingual	1/100-1/400 gr (150-600 μg); may repeat every 5 min ×2
(Nitrolingual)	Aerosol	1-2 metered doses; may repeat every 5 min ×2
(Nitrogard)	Prophylaxis: Extended release buccal tablets	1 mg q 5h
(Nitro-Bid, Nitrospan, Nitrong)	Extended release capsules	2.5, 6.5, or 9.0 mg q 8-12h
	Extended release tablets	1.3, 2.6, or 6.5 mg q 8-12h
(Nitrol)	Ointment	15-30 mg (1-2 inches) q 4h
	Maximum	75 mg (5 inches) per application
(Nitro-Dur, Nitrodisc, Transderm-Nitro)	Transdermal	1 unit (10-60 cm^2) qd
(Tridil)	Acute ischemia: Infusion	50 mg/500 ml D_5W (1 ml = 100 μg) at 5 μg/min; increase by 5 μg every 3-5 min; if no response at 20 μg, increase by 10 μg; titrate to patient relief of pain

Description

The nitrates have vasodilating effects predominantly in the venous circulation. They allow for peripheral pooling, decreased venous return to the heart, and reduced ventricular volume and pressure. Thus left ventricular wall tension (preload) is reduced, which decreases the demand for myocardial oxygen. Nitrates also reduce afterload via direct relaxation of vascular smooth muscle. Coronary blood flow and oxygen delivery are improved with coronary artery dilatation; therefore, myocardial ischemia is reduced.

Nitrates are used to treat angina and heart failure associated with acute MI. Major cardiovascular side effects include tachycardia and hypotension.

Nitrate tolerance, which affects the therapeutic efficacy of the drug, can develop with uninterrupted administration of long-acting nitrates. Tolerance does not seem to be a problem with short-acting nitrates, such as sublingual nitroglycerin.

Nitrates are available in many forms, allowing for various modes of administration. See Table 4-7 for a comparison of nitrates delivery dosage forms.

Clinical Alert

Concurrent administration of nitrates and other drugs that affect cardiovascular function can potentiate or antagonize the pharmacologic effects of these drugs.

Administration Precautions: Nitrates

- Do not administer to patients with hypertrophic cardiomyopathy who are experiencing chest pain, since angina may be aggravated.
- Do not administer to patients with cerebral hemorrhage or recent head trauma, since nitrates may increase cerebrospinal fluid pressure.
- Profound hypotension may occur in patients who are volume depleted.
- Monitor pulse; a 10 bpm increase is an indication of adequate vasodilation.
- Avoid abrupt termination of long-term or high-dosage nitrate therapy, since rebound angina may occur.
- If systolic blood pressure is <90 mm Hg or if the patient experiences dizziness or faints, do not administer the drug. Remove ointment or patch, or discontinue infusion.

Form	Use	Advantages	Disadvantages
Sublingual	Acute anginal attacks	Rapid onset; 1-4 min	Saliva needed to dissolve tablet; replacement is necessary 6 months after opening the bottle; protection from light and heat is necessary
Aerosol lingual	Acute anginal attacks	Rapid onset; not dependent on saliva for effectiveness; 3-year drug potency; not affected by heat or light	Shaking container causes an increase in propellant, resulting in less nitroglycerin delivered to patient
Oral*	Angina prophylaxis		Increased dosages are needed; orthostatic changes are more pronounced
Sustained release*	Angina prophylaxis	Constant amount of nitroglycerin is released over a longer duration	Not all products are equivalent
Topical ointment	Angina prophylaxis		Skin irritation; messy
Transdermal*	Angina prophylaxis	Dosage given only once a day; patient convenience	Skin irritation
IV*	Acute ischemia	Rapid onset (1-2 min); short duration (3-5 min)	

*Nitrate tolerance can develop.

- Avoid putting ointment on areas where defibrillator paddles or ECG electrodes are placed. Arc formation can result from defibrillation, and ointment alters the skin's electrical resistance.
- Remove transdermal patches before cardioversion to avoid formation of arcs.
- Intra-arterial monitoring is recommended when administering IV nitroglycerin. Monitor blood pressure every 3 to 5 minutes during IV titration; when chest pain is relieved and the patient is stabilized, monitor blood pressure every ½ to 1 hour.
- Intravenous nitroglycerin requires a glass container and specialized tubing (the drug can migrate into standard tubing and alter the calculated dosage to be delivered).
- Dosage schedules for long-acting nitrates should include a low-nitrate or nitrate-free period to prevent tolerance; transdermal patches and ointments should be removed after 12 to 14 hours.
- Moisture is required for sublingual tablets to dissolve rapidly.
- Buccal tablets should be placed between the upper lip and gum.
- Use the premeasured paper for ointment; rotate sites.
- Do not cut transdermal patches; avoid areas where cutaneous circulation is decreased; replace patch if it becomes loose or falls off.

Patient Assessment: Nitrates

- Evaluate for resolution of chest discomfort and decreased episodes of angina.
- Evaluate cardiac output (see Appendix C).
- See Reportable Adverse Effects, which follow.

Reportable Adverse Effects: Nitrates

- Unrelieved chest pain.
- Hypotension, dizziness, faintness.
- Blurred vision, dry mouth, severe headache.
- Signs of overdose: cyanotic lips, nailbeds, or palmar surface of hands; extreme dizziness, fainting, and feeling of pressure in the head; dyspnea, fever, seizure, weak or fast heart rate.

Calcium Channel Blocking Agents

The calcium channel blocking agents are summarized in Table 4-8.

Table 4-8 Calcium channel blocking agents

Drug	Indication and Usual Dosage	
Bepridil (Vascor)	Angina:	
	Oral	200 mg qd
	Maximum	400 mg qd
Diltiazem (Cardizem)	Angina:	
	Oral	30 mg tid-qid
	Maximum	360 mg qd
	Atrial fibrillation/flutter:	
	IV	0.25 mg/kg over 2 min; 0.35 mg/kg if inadequate response after 15 min of initial dose
	Infusion	5-15 mg/hr; do not exceed 24h of infusion
(Cardizem SR)	High blood pressure:	
	Oral	60-120 mg bid
	Maximum	360 mg qd
Felodipine (Plendil)	High blood pressure:	
	Oral	5 mg qd
	Maximum	20 mg qd
Isradipine (DynaCirc)	High blood pressure:	
	Oral	2.5 mg bid
	Maximum	20 mg qd
Nicardipine (Cardene)	Angina and high blood pressure:	
	Oral	20 mg q 8h
	Range	20-40 mg q 8h
Nifedipine (Procardia, Adalat)	Angina and high blood pressure:	
	Oral	10 mg tid
	Sublingual	10-20 mg
	Maximum	180 mg qd
(Procardia XL)	Oral	30 or 60 mg qd
(Adalat P.A.)	Oral	20 mg bid
Verapamil (Isoptin, Calan)	Dysrhythmias, high blood pressure, or angina:	
	Oral	80-120 mg tid initially
	Range	240-480 mg
	Sustained release	120-240 mg qd
	PAT/PSVT: IV	2.5-5 mg given over 2-3 min; repeat with 5-10 mg in 15-30 min (maximum 20 mg)

Continued.

Table 4-8   Calcium channel blocking agents—cont'd

Drug	Indication and Usual Dosage	
Verapamil—cont'd	High blood pressure:	
(Verelan)	Oral	240 mg qd
(Calan SR)	Oral	120-240 mg qd

Description

Calcium channel blocking agents prevent calcium from entering cells and consequently affect electrical activity of cardiac cells (calcium is necessary for phase two of the action potential), contraction of cardiac muscle, and vasomotor tone. Myocardial oxygen supply and demand are affected, making these agents useful in the treatment of angina. The vasodilating effect of these agents makes them useful in the treatment of high blood pressure and peripheral vascular disease. The depression of impulses from the SA node as well as the transmission of impulses through the AV node make verapamil particularly beneficial in treating select dysrhythmias. Nicardipine and nifedipine are more selective to vascular smooth muscle than cardiac muscle and have less effect on contractility and electrical conduction. Major cardiovascular side effects of calcium channel blockers are hypotension, bradycardia, sinus block, AV block, negative inotropic effect (heart failure), and reflex tachycardia (nifedipine, nicardipine).

Clinical Alert

Concurrent use of calcium channel blocking agents and other drugs that affect cardiovascular function may potentiate or antagonize the pharmacologic effects of these drugs.

Administration Precautions: Calcium Channel Blocking Agents

- Do not administer to patients with aortic stenosis; the decrease in diastolic pressure may worsen the myocardial oxygen supply and demand balance.
- Do not administer to patients in cardiogenic shock.
- Reduced dosages may be required in patients with impaired renal or hepatic function.
- Use cautiously in patients with heart failure, which may

worsen because of the drug's depressant effect.

- An increased risk for digitalis toxicity exists when patients take calcium channel blocking agents and digitalis concurrently.
- Check heart rate and blood pressure before drug administration; do not administer if systolic blood pressure <90 mm Hg, if dizziness or fainting occur, or if pulse <50 bpm.
- Gingival hyperplasia may develop.
- Development of pedal edema may be related to dosage.

Patient Assessment: Calcium Channel Blocking Agents

- Evaluate episodes of angina, blood pressure control, resolution or control of dysrhythmias.
- See Reportable Adverse Effects, which follow.

Reportable Adverse Effects: Calcium Channel Blocking Agents

- Chest pain, systolic blood pressure <90 mm Hg, heart rate <50 bpm, dysrhythmias, prolongation of PR interval, dizziness and fainting.
- Development or worsening of heart failure (S_3, crackles, fluid retention, shortness of breath, cough, or wheeze).

Administration Precautions: Specific Agents

Bepridil

- Can induce new dysrhythmias (i.e., VT/VF).
- Can prolong QT interval and cause torsades de pointes

Diltiazem

- Do not administer to patients with sinus node disease, advanced heart block, or Wolff-Parkinson-White (W-P-W) syndrome.
- Bradycardia and heart block can develop.
- Measure serial PR intervals.

Nicardipine

- Indicated in effort angina.
- Angina may increase with initial dosage.
- Measure blood pressure at intervals of 1 to 2 and 8 hours after dosing, during initial therapy, and during titration of the drug.

Nifedipine

- Use cautiously in cardiac patients, since reflex tachycardia can exacerbate angina.
- Capsules can be punctured to administer the drug sublingually or buccally.

Verapamil

- See diltiazem.
- Space IV administration of verapamil and beta adrenergic blocking agents a few hours apart to avoid profound cardiac-depressant effects.
- Withhold disopyramide 48 hours before and 24 hours after verapamil administration to avoid profound negative inotropic effects.

Antidysrhythmic Agents

Overview

The electrical cells of the heart possess the properties of automaticity (ability to generate an impulse), conductivity (ability to transmit the impulse), and excitability (ability to respond to an electrical impulse). Dysrhythmias are the result of a disturbance in impulse formation or impulse conduction and can adversely affect cardiac output. Antidysrhythmic agents act on the various phases of the action potential (Figure 4-1) to affect automaticity, conduction, and excitability of cardiac cells.

Although the goal of antidysrhythmic therapy is to abolish or control the disturbance, antidysrhythmic agents may be prodysrhythmic. In addition to heart block, changes in heart rate and other dysrhythmias can develop. A polymorphic form of ventricular tachycardia, known as torsades de pointes, can develop with the use of antidysrhythmic agents that prolong the QT interval.

The Vaughan-Williams classification has been used to group the antidysrhythmic agents into four classes (Table 4-9). Although each class consists of drugs with similar electrophysiologic properties, most antidysrhythmic agents share properties from other classes that are important to the overall antidysrhythmic efficacy of these drugs.

Digitalis is an antidysrhythmic agent used to treat atrial dysrhythmias and is discussed under cardiotonic agents later in this chapter. A summary of antidysrhythmic agents and their effects on cardiac function can be found in Table 4-10.

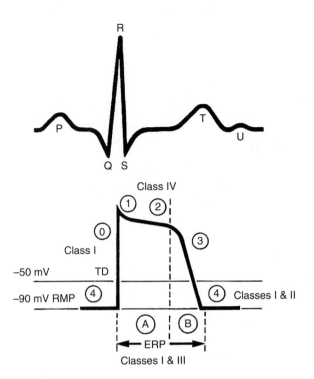

Figure 4-1

Antidysrhythmic agents and the cardiac action potential. The action potential consists of five phases: *Phase 0,* Depolarization of myocardium; rapid influx of sodium. *Phase 1,* Initial repolarization; sodium channels close. *Phase 2,* Plateau of repolarization; calcium enters the cell. *Phase 3,* Rapid repolarization; calcium channels close; potassium leaves the cell. *Phase 4,* Resting phase; sodium-potassium pump is removing sodium from the cell and returning potassium into the cell to restore the ionic balance. Phases 0 to 3 correlate with systole; phase 4 correlates with diastole. *TP,* Threshold potential, the level at which excitation of cardiac muscle occurs; *RMP,* Resting membrane potential, the level at which ionic balance is restored; *ERP,* Effective refractory period, a period of decreased excitability. **A,** Absolute refractory period; **B,** relative refractory period.

Table 4-9 Electrophysiologic effects of antidysrhythmic agents

Class	Electrophysiologic Effects
I Membrane stabilizing agents; sodium channel blockers (local anesthetics)	Slow upstroke of phase 0; decrease excitability; slow conduction velocity; suppress automaticity in ectopic pacemakers
IA Disopyramide Procainamide Quinidine	Moderately slow upstroke of phase 0; prolong action potential duration; decrease excitability; slow conduction velocity
IB Lidocaine Mexiletine Phenytoin Tocainide	Slightly slow upstroke of phase 0; shorten the action potential in normal fibers
IC Encainide Flecainide Propafenone* Moricizine	Markedly slow upstroke of phase 0; no effect on action potential duration; slow conduction velocity
II Beta adrenergic blocking agents Acebutolol Esmolol Propranolol	Depress phase 4 in sinus node; slow AV nodal conduction velocity; block effects of sympathetic tone on the heart
III Agents that prolong repolarization Amiodarone Bretylium	Prolong action potential duration; have antifibrillatory effect
IV Calcium channel blocking agents Verapamil	Depresses phase 4 depolarization; prolongs phase 2 of repolarization

*Has properties of IA, IB, and IC subclasses.

Table 4-10   **Summary of the effects of antidysrhythmic drugs on cardiac function**

	Automaticity	ERP	Contractility	PR Interval	QT Interval
IA	↓	↑	↓	↑	↑
IB	↓	↓	0	0	0/↓
IC	↓	↑	0	↑	↑
II	↓	0/↓	↓	↑	0
III	↓	↑	↓	↑	↑
IV	↓	↑	↓	↑	0

IA, Disopyramide, Procainamide, Quinidine, IB, Lidocaine, Mexiletine, Phenytoin, Tocainide. IC, Encainide, Flecainide, Propafenone, Moricizine. II, Acebutolol, Esmolol, Propranolol. III, Amiodarone, Bretylium. IV, Verapamil. ERP, Effective refractory period. ↑, increase. ↓, decrease. 0, no effect.

Class IA Antidysrhythmic Agents

Class IA antidysrhythmic agents are summarized in Table 4-11.

Description

Class IA antidysrhythmic agents are membrane-active drugs that block the influx of sodium and depress phase 0 of the action potential. Automaticity, conductivity, and contractility are reduced. In addition, the effective refractory period is prolonged. These agents also block parasympathetic nerve impulses to the SA and AV node, thereby increasing the conduction rate of the AV node. Class IA agents are used to treat both atrial and ventricular dysrhythmias. Major cardiovascular side effects include dysrhythmias, increased ventricular rates, hypotension, negative inotropic effect (heart failure), and prolonged QT interval.

Clinical Alert

Concurrent administration of class IA antidysrhythmic agents and other drugs that affect cardiovascular function can potentiate or antagonize the pharmacologic effects of these drugs.

Administration Precautions: Class IA Agents

- Do not administer class IA agents to patients with advanced AV block; measure PR intervals.

Table 4-11   Class IA antidysrhythmic agents

Drug	Indication and Usual Dosage	
Disopyramide phosphate (Norpace)	Ventricular dysrhythmias:	
	Oral	300 mg loading dose
	Maintenance	150 mg q 6h
	Extended-release form	300 mg q 12h
Procainamide (Pronestyl)	Atrial dysrhythmias:	
	Oral	1.25 g initially; 750 mg 1 hour later if needed; 500-1000 mg q 2-3h
	Sustained release	1000 mg q 6h
	Ventricular dysrhythmias:	
	Oral	1 g initially; then 50 mg/kg/day in 8 divided doses
	Sustained release	50 mg/kg/day in 4 divided doses
	IV	20 mg/min until dysrhythmia is abolished; hypotension occurs; QRS widens by 50%; or a total of 17 mg/kg has been given.
	Infusion	2 g/500 ml D_5W (1 ml = 4 mg); at 1-4 mg/min
Quinidine sulfate	Atrial fibrillation:	
	Oral	200 mg q 2-3h (for 5-8 doses)
	Maintenance	200-300 mg 3-4×/day
(Quinidex exten-tabs)	Oral	300 or 600 mg q 8-12h
Quinidine Gluconate (Quinaglute Dura-tabs)	Oral	324-660 mg q 6-12h

- Prolonged QT interval can occur; these agents should be discontinued when the QRS complex widens or QT interval lengthens by greater than 25%. Measure serial QT intervals.
- Use cautiously in patients with hepatic or renal impairment.
- Atrial fibrillation or atrial flutter should be treated with digitalis before administering these agents to avoid the risk of tachycardia.
- Administer these agents at equally spaced intervals.

Patient Assessment: Class IA Agents

- Evaluate dysrhythmia control.
- Evaluate cardiac output status (see Appendix C).
- See Reportable Adverse Effects for specific agents.

Administration Precautions: Specific Agents

Disopyramide

- Do not administer to patients in heart failure; this agent is a cardiac depressant.
- Do not administer 48 hours before or 24 hours after verapamil; deaths have occurred.
- Wait 6 to 12 hours to administer disopyramide if patient has received quinidine and 3 to 6 hours if patient has received procainamide.
- Hypoglycemia may result in patients with heart failure or hepatic or renal impairment or in patients taking certain drugs such as beta blockers, insulin, or oral antidiabetic agents.

Procainamide

- Do not exceed an intravenous rate of 20 mg/min; severe hypotension, reflex tachycardia, ventricular fibrillation, and asystole may result.
- Use cautiously in patients with lupus erythematosus; the condition may be exacerbated.

Quinidine

- Concurrent use with digitalis can increase risk for digitalis toxicity.
- Use cautiously in patients with myasthenia gravis, since increased weakness can occur.

Reportable Adverse Effects: Specific Agents

Disopyramide

- Inability to void.
- Hypotension, signs of decreased cardiac output, irregular heart rhythm, and heart failure.
- Signs of hypoglycemia.
- Widened QRS complex, prolonged QT interval, and torsades de pointes.

Procainamide

- Joint pain, fever, and chills (SLE-type signs and symptoms).
- Widened QRS complex, prolonged PR and QT intervals and torsades de pointes.
- Heart failure, hypotension.
- Agranulocytosis, thrombocytopenia, and elevated ANA titer.
- Signs of overdosage include confusion, dizziness, decrease in urination, nausea and vomiting, tachycardia or irregular heart rhythm.

Quinidine

- Widened QRS complex, prolonged PR and QT intervals, and torsades de pointes.
- Thrombocytopenia.
- Cinchonism (blurred vision, headache, nausea, and tinnitus).
- Signs of toxicity include syncope, hypotension, dysrhythmias (ventricular ectopy or tachycardia).

Class IB Antidysrhythmic Agents

Class IB antidysrhythmic agents are summarized in Table 4-12.

Description

Class IB agents block sodium from entering the cell during phase 0 of the action potential. They decrease automaticity and the action potential duration in Purkinje fibers and ventricular cells. Lidocaine is administered intravenously only and is the first-line drug used for immediate treatment of life-threatening ventricular dysrhythmias. Tocainide and mexiletine are oral preparations used to treat patients with chronic ventricular dysrhythmias. Phenytoin is used in the treatment of dysrhythmias caused by digitalis toxicity.

Table 4-12   Class IB antidysrhythmic agents

Drug	Indication and Usual Dosage	
Lidocaine (Xylocaine)	Ventricular dysrhythmia:	
	IV bolus	1-1.5 mg/kg; repeat 0.5-1.5 mg/kg every 5-10 minutes (up to 3 mg/kg)
	Infusion	2 g/500 ml D_5W (1 ml = 4 mg); at 2-4 mg/min
Mexiletine (Mexitil)	Ventricular dysrhythmia:	
	Oral	400 mg loading dose; 200 mg q 8h
Phenytoin (Dilantin)	Digitalis induced dysrhythmia:	
	IV	100 mg every 5 min (but no more than 50 mg/min) until effective, 1000 mg have been given, or toxic effects are observed
	Oral	Day 1: 1000 mg; days 2 and 3: 500 mg; 300-500 mg qd maintenance dose
Tocainide (Tonocard)	Ventricular dysrhythmia:	
	Oral	400 mg q 8h

Major cardiovascular side effects of class IB antidysrhythmic agents include hypotension and bradycardia.

Clinical Alert

Concurrent use of class IB antidysrhythmic agents and other drugs that affect cardiovascular function can potentiate or antagonize the pharmacologic effects of these drugs.

Administration Precautions: Class IB Agents

- These agents are contraindicated in patients with advanced heart block; measure serial PR intervals.
- Use cautiously in patients with liver or renal impairment.

Patient Assessment: Class IB Agents

- Evaluate dysrhythmia control.
- Evaluate cardiac output (see Appendix C).
- See Reportable Adverse Effects for specific agents.

Administration Precautions: Specific Agents

Lidocaine

- Not recommended in patients with atrial flutter or ventricular escape beats.
- A loading dose and infusion control device is required with lidocaine administration.
- Incidence of adverse effects increases in the elderly population.

Mexiletine

- May precipitate seizures.
- If replacing other antidysrhythmic agents, initiate mexiletine 6 to 12 hours after the last dose of quinidine or dysopyramide; 3 to 6 hours after procainamide; 8 to 12 hours after tocainide.

Phenytoin

- Do not mix IV phenytoin with any other drug; administer normal saline after IV use to reduce vessel irritation and prevent any drug precipitation.
- Do not administer >50 mg/min; death from cardiac arrest has occurred after too rapid IV injection.

Tocainide

- Onset of trembling or shaking may be a sign that maximum dosage has been achieved.
- Pulmonary fibrosis or toxicity may develop.

Reportable Adverse Effects: Specific Agents

Lidocaine

- Confusion, agitation, slurred speech, dysarthria, paresthesia, tinnitus, tremors, twitching, seizures, and coma.
- Dysrhythmias.

Mexiletine

- Same effects as lidocaine.
- Blood dyscrasias.
- Dysrhythmias.
- Fever, chills, sore throat, and bleeding.

Phenytoin

- Hypotension, bradycardia, and heart block.
- Confusion, nystagmus, tremors, and visual disturbances.

Tocainide

- Same effects as lidocaine.
- Blood dyscrasias.
- Cough, shortness of breath.
- Fever, chills, sore throat, and bleeding.

Class IC Antidysrhythmic Agents

Class IC antidysrhythmic agents are summarized in Table 4-13.

Description

Class IC antidysrhythmic agents act on the cell membrane by blocking sodium channels. They decrease automaticity, conduction velocity, and excitability in Purkinje fibers. These agents are used to treat life-threatening dysrhythmias such as sustained ventricular tachycardia.

Clinical Alert

Concurrent administration of class IC antidysrhythmic agents and other drugs that affect cardiovascular function may potentiate or antagonize the pharmacologic effects of these drugs.

Administration Precautions: Class IC Agents

- Do not give to patients with advanced AV heart block or right bundle branch block with a hemiblock. Measure serial PR intervals.
- Electrolyte imbalances should be corrected before these agents are administered.
- Use cautiously in patients with renal or hepatic impairment, congestive heart failure, or prolonged QT interval. Measure serial QT intervals.

Table 4-13   Class IC antidysrhythmic agents

Drug	Usual Dosage	
Encainide (Enkaid)	Oral	25 mg q8h
	Maximum	50 mg q6h
Flecainide (Tambocor)	Oral	100 mg q12h
Moricizine (Ethmozine)	Oral	200-300 mg q8h
Propafenone (Rhythmol)	Oral	150 mg q8h

- Use cautiously in patients with pacemakers. Class IC agents increase the endocardial pacing threshold and may suppress ventricular escape rhythms. Determine pacing threshold periodically in patients with pacemakers.
- Not recommended for mild or moderate heart rhythm irregularities.
- Encainide and flecainide are associated with excessive mortality or increased nonfatal cardiac arrest rate in patients who recently experienced MI and have asymptomatic non-life-threatening dysrhythmias. During the development and testing of moricizine, some deaths occurred in patients with life-threatening ventricular dysrhythmias.

Patient Assessment: Class IC Agents

- Evaluate dysrhythmia control.
- Evaluate cardiac output (see Appendix C).
- See Reportable Adverse Effects, which follow.

Reportable Adverse Effects: Class IC Agents

- Dysrhythmias.
- Heart failure, chest pain.
- QT prolongation, QRS widening.
- Hypotension, seizures.

Class II Antidysrhythmic Agents

See discussion under Beta Adrenergic Blocking Agents (p. 166).

Class III Antidysrhythmic Agents

Class III antidysrhythmic agents are summarized in Table 4-14.

Description

Class III antidysrhythmic agents prolong the action potential duration. Automaticity of ventricular ectopic areas is depressed. The specific mechanism for bretylium is unknown but is thought to suppress ventricular tachycardia by depleting norepinephrine stores and inhibiting release of norepinephrine. Amiodarone has a negative inotropic effect and produces peripheral and coronary artery vasodilation. Major cardiovascular side effects of Class III agents include orthostatic hypotension, dysrhythmias, bradycardia, and angina.

Table 4-14   Class III antidysrhythmic agents

Drug	Indication and Usual Dosage	
Amiodarone (Cordarone)	Ventricular dysrhythmias:	
	Oral	800-1600 mg (loading dose) qd for 1-3 weeks; 600 mg qd for 4 weeks; 400 mg qd or may alternate with 600 mg
	IV	5 mg/kg over 20 min to 2 hours
Bretylium (Bretylol)	Ventricular fibrillation:	
	IV	5 mg/kg; defibrillate; increase to 10 mg/kg and repeat every 5 min to the maximum of 30-35 mg/kg
	Ventricular tachycardia:	
	IV	5-10 mg/kg diluted to 50 ml with D_5W can be injected over 8-10 min
	Infusion	2 g/500 ml D_5W (1 ml = 4 mg); at 2 mg/min

Clinical Alert

Concurrent administration of class III antidysrhythmic agents and other drugs that affect cardiovascular function may potentiate or antagonize the pharmacologic effects of these drugs.

Administration Precautions: Specific Agents

Amiodarone

· Do not administer to patients with AV block, bradycardia with syncope, or sinus node dysfunction. Measure serial PR intervals.
· Measure serial QT intervals.
· Pulmonary toxicity may develop.
· Hepatic dysfunction may develop.
· Elimination is slow; thus amiodarone can interact with other pharmacologic agents months after discontinuation.

Bretylium

· Contraindicated in patients with digitalis-induced dysrhythmias.
· Correct hypovolemia before administering.

- Patient may experience hypertension with initial administration because of the initial release of norepinephrine; hypotension follows.
- Keep patient supine during infusion.
- Monitor blood pressure frequently during infusion.
- Rapid IV administration may cause nausea or vomiting.

Patient Assessment: Class III Agents

- Evaluate dysrhythmia control.
- Evaluate cardiac output (see Appendix C).
- See Reportable Adverse Effects, which follow.

Reportable Adverse Effects: Specific Agents

Amiodarone

- Adventitious breath sounds; difficulty breathing.
- Dysrhythmias.
- Signs of hyperthyroidism (weight loss, insomnia, nervousness, sensitivity to heat, and sweating) or hypothyroidism (weight gain, coldness, tiredness, and dry skin).
- Difficulty walking, trembling, shaking, numbness, photophobia, blurred vision, blue-gray skin tone, heart failure, and epididymitis.

Bretylium

- Dysrhythmias.
- Hypotension, dizziness, and syncope.
- Angina.

Class IV Antidysrhythmic Agents

See discussion on Calcium Blocking Agents (p. 174).

Other Antidysrhythmic Agent

Description

Adenosine (Adenocard) restores normal sinus rhythm by slowing conduction time through the AV node. Adenosine is used to treat paroxysmal supraventricular tachycardia (PVST) including PSVT associated with Wolff-Parkinson-White syndrome. (See the box on p. 191 for administration.)

Adenosine (Adenocard)

Administer 6 mg IV bolus over 1-2 sec (slow administration may result in ↑ HR in response to vasodilatation).

Flush IV with saline to assure drug reaches the circulatory system.

Wait 1-2 minutes.

If conversion to sinus rhythm is unsuccessful, give 12 mg rapidly IV.

Repeat the 12 mg dose if necessary.

Discard any unused solution.

Administration Precautions: Adenosine

· Use cautiously in patients with asthma because inhaled adenosine causes bronchoconstriction.
· A short-lasting first-, second-, or third-degree heart block may result (half-life of adenosine is <10 seconds).
· New dysrhythmias may develop during conversion (PVCs, PACs, bradycardia, tachycardia, AV block).
· Use cautiously in patients receiving dipyridamole or carbamazepine since both drugs potentiate the effects of adenosine; higher degrees of heart block may result with carbamazepine.
· Use cautiously in patients receiving theophylline or other methylxanthine products, since the effects of adenosine are antagonized by methylxanthines.

Patient Assessment: Adenosine

· Evaluate heart rate and rhythm 1 to 2 minutes after administering adenosine.
· Monitor blood pressure; large doses may cause hypotension.
· Measure PR interval for development of AV block.
· See Reportable Adverse Effects, which follow.

Reportable Adverse Effects: Adenosine

· Hypotension, dyspnea, nonmyocardial chest discomfort.
· Facial flushing, sweating, headache, tingling in arms, blurred vision, numbness, heaviness in arms, burning sensation, neck and back pain, metallic taste, tightness in throat, pressure in groin.

Cardiotonic Agents

Overview

Cardiotonic agents such as cardiac glycosides and phosphodiesterase inhibitors are used to improve myocardial contractility. The improved inotropic state of the failing heart results in an increase in cardiac output. The improved output enhances blood flow to the kidneys, which explains the diuretic effect often associated with these agents.

Cardiac Glycoside Agents

Table 4-15 lists these agents and usual dosages.

Description

These agents inhibit sodium potassium ATPase, which causes an increase in cellular calcium influx. This increased concentration of calcium is responsible for the increase in contractility, which makes these agents beneficial in the treatment of heart failure. Cardiac glycosides also increase the refractory period of the SA and AV nodes and decrease conductivity. They are therefore useful in treating atrial dysrhythmias. The major cardiovascular side effect is digitalis toxicity (see the box on p. 193).

Clinical Alert

Concurrent use of digitalis preparations and drugs that affect cardiovascular function may potentiate or antagonize the pharmacologic effects of these drugs.

Table 4-15   **Cardiac glycoside agents**

Drug	Indication and Usual Dosage	
Digoxin	Oral digitalization	0.4-1 mg
(Lanoxin)	IV digitalization	0.5-0.75 mg
	Maintenance	IV/PO 0.125-0.5 mg qd
Digitoxin	Oral digitalization	1.2-1.6 mg in divided doses
(Crystodigin)	IV digitalization	1.0-1.6 mg in divided doses
	Maintenance	0.10 mg qd

Administration Precautions: Cardiac Glycoside Agents

- Digitalis preparations have prodysrhythmic effects.
- Patients with partial AV block may develop complete heart block; measure serial PR intervals.
- Patients with Wolff-Parkinson-White syndrome may experience fatal ventricular dysrhythmias.
- Patients who have taken digitalis preparations in the previous 2 to 3 weeks should receive reduced dosages for digitalization.
- The risk of digitalis toxicity (see box below) is increased in the elderly and in those with impaired renal function.
- Do not administer if apical pulse is <60 bpm.

𝒶 Digitalis Toxicity

Signs and Symptoms

Loss of appetite
Nausea or vomiting
Stomach pain
Unusual fatigue
Slowed heart rate
Dysrhythmias (sinus bradycardia, sinus arrest, AV block, PVCs, PAT with block, AV dissociation, junctional rhythms, ventricular tachycardia)
Vision disturbances (yellow, green, or white halos)
Confusion, drowsiness, headache, and irritability
ST segment sagging and prolonged PR interval

Treatment

Discontinue digitalis
Temporary pacemaker may be needed
Correct electrolyte imbalance
Administer phenytoin sodium (Dilantin) for atrial, junctional, or ventricular tachycardia
Avoid quinidine when treating dysrhythmias because it increases serum digitalis levels
Administer intravenous digoxin immune Fab (Digibind) in a dosage equimolar to the amount of digitalis in the body; 40 mg of Digibind = 0.6 mg of digoxin or digitoxin

- Electrolyte imbalances and other factors can alter the effectiveness of digoxin (see box below); check electrolyte levels.
- Be prepared to administer potassium chloride if the patient is hypokalemic. Intravenous potassium should never be administered undiluted and should not exceed a rate of 20 mEq/hour unless severe hypokalemia exists. The patient's ECG should be monitored during potassium infusion.
- Wait at least 6 hours after the last oral dose and at least 4 hours after the last IV dose to draw blood for serum digoxin levels.

Patient Assessment: Cardiac Glycoside Agents

- Assess for resolution of heart failure or controlled atrial fibrillation or atrial flutter (decreased ventricular response).
- See Reportable Adverse Effects, which follow.

Select Factors Affecting Digoxin Effectiveness

Drugs that Increase Risk for Toxicity

Amiodarone
Antacids
Quinidine
Calcium channel blockers
Diuretics
Steroids
Amphotericin B

Electrolyte Imbalances that Increase Risk for Toxicity

Hypokalemia
Hypomagnesemia
Hypercalcemia

Conditions that Increase Risk for Toxicity

Hepatic impairment
Renal impairment
Hypothyroidism

Drugs that Decrease Digoxin Bioavailability

Antacids
Cholestyramine
Neomycin

Reportable Adverse Effects: Cardiac Glycoside Agents

- Signs and symptoms of digitalis toxicity (see box on p. 193).
- Apical pulse <60 bpm.
- Elevated serum digoxin level (see Appendix F).

Phosphodiesterase Inhibitors

The phosphodiesterase inhibitors are summarized in Table 4-16.

Description

These nonglycoside, noncatecholamine, cardiotonic agents are used in treating congestive heart failure. They exert a positive inotropic effect by inhibiting myocardial cyclic adenosine monophosphate (cAMP) phosphodiesterase activity and increase cellular cAMP. These agents also possess vasodilator properties that reduce after-load and preload, contributing to improved left ventricular function without increasing myocardial oxygen demand. Milrinone is more potent than amrinone. The major cardiovascular side effects of amrinone include dysrhythmias, hypotension, and chest pain.

Clinical Alert

Concurrent use of amrinone and other drugs that affect cardiovascular function may potentiate or antagonize the pharmacologic effects of these drugs.

Table 4-16   Phosphodiesterase inhibitors

Drug		Usual Dosage
Amrinone (Inocor)	IV	750 μg/kg over 2-3 min then
	Infusion	100 mg/100 ml NS (1 ml-1000 μg) at 5-15 μg/kg/min
	Maximum	18 μg/kg/min
Milrinone (Corotrope)	IV	50 μg/kg over 10 min, then
	Infusion	0.375 μg/kg/min
(Primacor)	IV	50 μg/kg over 10 min, then
	Infusion	0.5 μg/kg/min

Administration Precautions: Phosphodiesterase Inhibitors

- Contraindications include hypertrophic cardiomyopathy, acute MI, severe aortic/pulmonic valvular disease.
- Avoid concomitant administration with disopyramide (Norpace).
- Digitalis is recommended in patients with atrial flutter or fibrillation, since amrinone can increase ventricular response.
- Use cautiously in patients with hepatic and renal impairment.
- Hypotension may result from amrinone administration.
- Thrombocytopenia may occur; platelet counts should be done before and during amrinone therapy.
- Do not mix amrinone with dextrose solutions.

Patient Assessment: Phosphodiesterase Inhibitors

- Monitor blood pressure and other hemodynamic parameters (CVP, PAWP, CI, CO) frequently during amrinone infusion.
- Assess other parameters of cardiac output status (see Appendix C).
- See Reportable Adverse Effects, which follow.

Reportable Adverse Effects: Phosphodiesterase Inhibitors

- Hypotension, dizziness, dysrhythmias, and chest pain.
- Hypokalemia, increased liver function values, and decreased platelet count.

Diuretic Agents

Overview

Diuretics rid the body of excess fluid, a major concern in patients with heart disease. When cardiac output falls, blood flow to the kidneys is decreased, which activates the renin-angiotensin-aldosterone system (Figure 4-2). This leads to an increase in blood pressure and preload, which does not necessarily increase the stroke volume. The increase in preload in heart failure can cause a further reduction in cardiac output. Diuretics reduce preload by promoting the excretion of sodium and water at various sites in the nephron (see Figure 4-3) and thus reduce the workload of the heart.

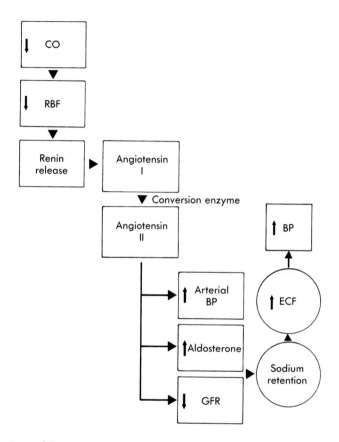

Figure 4-2
Renin-angiotensin-aldosterone system. *CO,* Cardiac output; *RBF,* renal blood flow; *BP,* blood pressure; *GFR,* glomerular filtration rate; *ECF,* extracellular fluid.

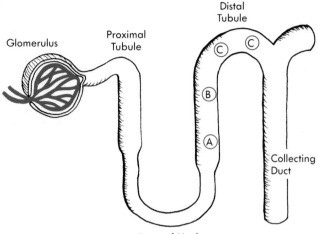

Figure 4-3
Nephron and sites of diuretic action. **A,** Loop diuretics (etha-crynic acid, furosemide, bumetanide). **B,** Thiazide diuretics (chlorthalidone, metolazone, indapamide). **C,** Potassium-sparing diuretics (spironolactone, triamterene, amiloride).

Thiazide and Thiazide-Like Diuretic Agents

See Table 4-17 for information on these agents.

Description

These agents increase sodium and water excretion by inhibiting so-dium reabsorption in the cortical thick ascending loop and distal convoluted tubules, thus reducing extracellular fluid and plasma volume. They also increase potassium, chloride, magnesium, and bicarbonate ion excretion. These agents are used to treat high blood pressure, edematous states, and congestive heart failure. Major car-diovascular side effects include orthostatic hypotension, volume depletion, and hypokalemia.

Clinical Alert

Concurrent use of diuretic agents and other drugs that affect car-diovascular function may potentiate or antagonize the pharmaco-logic effects of these drugs.

⚔ Table 4-17   Thiazide and thiazide-like diuretic agents

Drug	Indication and Usual Dosage
Chlorothiazide (Diuril)	Edematous states: Oral 500-1500 mg/day Hypertension: Oral 250-1000 mg/day
Chlorthalidone (Hygroton)	Edematous states or hypertension: Oral 25-100 mg qd
Metolazone (Zaroxolyn)	Edematous states: Oral 5-20 mg qd Hypertension: Oral 2.5-5 mg qd
Hydrochlorothiazide (Esidrix, Oretic, Hydro-Diuril)	Edematous states or hypertension: Oral 25-100 mg qd
Indapamide (Lozol)	Edematous states or hypertension: Oral 2.5 mg qd

Select Combination Agents

Aldactazide = spironolactone 25/50 mg and hydrochlorothiazide 25/50 mg

Capozide = captopril 25/50 mg and hydrochlorothiazide 15/25 mg

Diazide = triamterene 50 mg and hydrochlorothiazide 25 mg

Maxzide = triamterene 75 mg and hydrochlorothiazide 50 mg

Moduretic = amiloride 5 mg and hydrochlorothiazide 50 mg

Vaseretic = enalapril maleate 10 mg and hydrochlorothiazide 25mg

Zestoretic = lisinopril 20 mg and hydrochlorothiazide 12.5 or 25 mg

Administration Precautions: Thiazide and Thiazide-Like Agents

- Use cautiously in patients with renal disease.
- Hypovolemia may occur.
- Electrolyte imbalances, increased serum lipid levels, and increased blood urea nitrogen levels may occur.

- Diabetic patients may experience carbohydrate intolerance.
- Patients taking digoxin are at risk for hypokalemia and related digitalis toxicity.

Patient Assessment: Thiazide and Thiazide-Like Agents

- Evaluate fluid volume status (see Table 2-8).
- Evaluate blood pressure control.
- See Reportable Adverse Effects, which follow.

Reportable Adverse Effects: Thiazide and Thiazide-Like Agents

- Hypovolemia (see Table 2-8).
- Hypokalemia (see Table 4-18), glucose intolerance, hypercalcemia, hypophosphatemia, hyperuricemia, and metabolic alkalosis.

Loop Diuretic Agents

See Table 4-19 for information on loop diuretic agents.

Description

These agents are the most potent diuretics available. Loop diuretic agents inhibit sodium and chloride reabsorption in the thick ascending limb of the loop of Henle. Potassium, magnesium, calcium, and bicarbonate ions are excreted in addition to sodium and chloride. These agents are used to treat high blood pressure, edematous states, and congestive heart failure (CHF). Their major cardiovascular side effects include orthostatic hypotension, volume depletion, hypokalemia, and other electrolyte disturbances.

Table 4-18   Signs and symptoms of electrolyte imbalances

Hyponatremia	
Gastrointestinal	Abdominal cramps, anorexia, nausea, and vomiting
Neuromuscular	Fatigue, apathy, headache, muscle weakness or twitching, convulsions, and coma
Laboratory	Serum sodium <135 mEq/L
	Serum osmolality <285 mOsm/kg

Table 4-18   Signs and symptoms of electrolyte imbalances—cont'd

Hypokalemia	
Cardiovascular	Bradycardia; depressed ST segment; flattened, inverted T waves; U waves; dysrhythmias; cardiac arrest
Gastrointestinal	Abdominal distention, anorexia, nausea, vomiting, diarrhea, paralytic ileus
Neuromuscular	Fatigue, muscle weakness, paresthesias, lethargy, confusion, muscle cramps
Laboratory	Serum potassium <3.5 mEq/L
Hyperkalemia	
Cardiovascular	Peaked T waves, depressed ST segment, prolonged PR interval, widened QRS complex, ventricular ectopy, bradycardia, heart block, cardiac arrest
Gastrointestinal	Nausea, diarrhea, vomiting
Neuromuscular	Muscle twitching to paralysis, muscle weakness, numbness and tingling of face, tongue, hands, and feet
Laboratory	Serum potassium >5.5 mEq/L
Hypomagnesemia	
Neuromuscular	Confusion, agitation, convulsions, tremors, muscle cramps, increased reflexes, positive Chvostek's sign, positive Trousseau's sign
Cardiovascular	Tachycardia, tachydysrhythmias, prolonged PR interval, prolonged QT interval, widened QRS complex, ST segment depression, T wave inversion, hypotension
Laboratory	Serum magnesium <1.5 mEq/L
Hypocalcemia	
	Similar to hypomagnesemia
	Serum calcium <8.5 mg/dl

Table 4-19   Loop diuretic agents

Drug		Usual Dosage
Bumetanide (Bumex)	Oral	0.5-2 mg qd
	IV	0.5-1 mg
	Maximum	10 mg qd
Ethacrynic acid (Edecrin)	Oral	50-200 mg qd
	IV	0.5-1.0 mg/kg (not to exceed 100 mg in a single dose)
Furosemide (Lasix)	Oral	20-80 mg qd
	IV	20-40 mg

Clinical Alert

Concurrent administration of diuretics and other drugs that affect cardiovascular function may potentiate or antagonize the pharmacologic effects of these drugs.

Administration Precautions: Loop Diuretic Agents

- Use cautiously in patients with renal, hepatic, and pancreatic impairment.
- Severe electrolyte imbalances and volume depletion can occur.
- Patients receiving digoxin and diuretics are at increased risk for digitalis toxicity.
- Patients taking aspirin should be monitored for salicylate toxicity.
- Concurrent use of aminoglycosides and loop diuretics may cause ototoxicity.
- Combining lithium therapy with furosemide therapy can result in lithium toxicity.
- Serum lipid levels may increase.
- Impaired glucose tolerance can occur in diabetic patients.
- Rapid injection of furosemide may cause transient deafness.
- Lupus erythematosus may be exacerbated with furosemide or ethacrynic acid therapy.

Patient Assessment: Loop Diuretic Agents

- Evaluate blood pressure control.
- Evaluate fluid volume status (see Table 2-8).
- See Reportable Adverse Effects, which follow.

Reportable Adverse Effects: Loop Diuretic Agents

- Furosemide toxicity: tinnitus, abdominal pain, sore throat, and fever.
- Volume depletion (see Table 2-8).
- Hypokalemia, hyponatremia, hypochloremia, hypocalcemia, hypomagnesemia, hyperuricemia, metabolic alkalosis and impaired glucose tolerance.

Potassium Sparing Diuretic Agents

Table 4-20 lists these agents, indications, and usual dosages.

Description

Potassium sparing agents produce a diuretic effect without depleting potassium ions. These agents impair the exchange of sodium for potassium at the distal tubule to increase the excretion of sodium and conserve potassium, while also increasing the excretion of chloride and calcium ions. They are commonly used with other diuretics to minimize potassium loss and alkalosis. Potassium sparing agents are used to treat high blood pressure, edematous states, and CHF. Major cardiovascular side effects include hypotension, volume depletion, hyperkalemia, and other electrolyte disturbances.

Clinical Alert

Concurrent use of diuretic agents and other drugs that affect cardiovascular function may potentiate or antagonize the pharmacologic effects of these drugs.

Table 4-20 Potassium-sparing diuretic agents

Drug	Indication and Usual Dosage	
Amiloride (Midamor)	Edematous states or hypertension:	
	Oral	5-20 mg qd
Spironolactone (Aldactone)	Edematous states:	
	Oral	25-200 mg qd
	Hypertension:	
	Oral	50-100 mg qd
Triamterene (Dyrenium)	Edematous states:	
	Oral	25-300 mg qd

Administration Precautions: Potassium Sparing Diuretic Agents

- Contraindicated in patients with anuria and hyperkalemia.
- Exercise caution in administering to elderly or diabetic patients because renal function may be decreased.

Patient Assessment: Potassium Sparing Diuretic Agents

- Evaluate fluid volume status (see Table 2-8).
- Evaluate blood pressure control.
- See Reportable Adverse Effects, which follow.

Reportable Adverse Effects: Potassium Sparing Diuretic Agents

- Volume depletion (see Table 2-8).
- Hyperkalemia and hyponatremia (see Table 4-18).

Antihypertensive Agents

Overview

High blood pressure damages the heart and can affect other organs as well (see hypertension in Chapter 1). Patients can be treated with a combination of antihypertensive drugs in an attempt to control high blood pressure. Nonpharmacologic interventions such as weight loss and restriction of sodium should also be employed.

Antihypertensive agents are classified into many categories based on their mechanisms of action. These classifications are compared in Table 4-21. The sites of action of these agents are illustrated in Figure 4-4.

Some antihypertensive agents have a detrimental effect on serum lipid levels. Alpha adrenergic blockers, ACE inhibitors, and calcium channel blockers, however, have either a beneficial effect or no effect on serum lipid levels. Other cardiovascular side effects include hypotension, dysrhythmias, chest pain, and palpitations.

Alpha Adrenergic Blocking and Centrally Acting Agents

Alpha adrenergic blocking agents and centrally-acting agents are listed in Table 4-22.

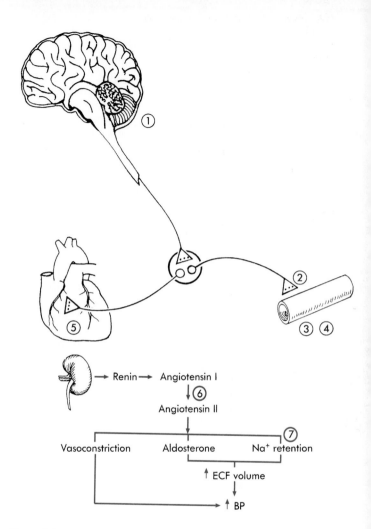

Figure 4-4
Sites of action of antihypertensive agents. 1, Centrally-acting agents depress sympathetic tone. 2, Alpha-adrenergic blocking agents block receptor sites. 3, Vasodilators dilate smooth muscle. 4, Calcium channel blocking agents dilate smooth muscle. 5, Beta-adrenergic blocking agents decrease cardiac output. 6, ACE inhibitors interfere with angiotensin II formation. 7, Diuretic agents block sodium reabsorption.

From Clark JB, Queener SF, Karb VB: *Pharmacological basis of nursing practice,* ed 4, St Louis, 1992, Mosby.

Table 4-21   Comparison of antihypertensive agents

Classification	Effect	Comment
Alpha adrenergic blocking agents	Decrease afterload, decrease preload	Predispose patients to symptomatic orthostatic hypotension.
Centrally acting alpha blockers	Decrease peripheral resistance with minimal effect on cardiac output (CO)	Diuretic agents are usually required.
Beta adrenergic blocking agents	Decrease CO and inhibit renin secretion	May cause bronchospasm in obstructive lung disease; may be used cautiously in patients with peripheral vascular disease and diabetes; may be beneficial in patients with rapid heart rates and increased pulse pressure.
Diuretics	Decrease preload, decrease afterload	Electrolyte alterations increase the risk for dysrhythmias; hyperglycemia and hypercholesterolemia are associated with long-term therapy.
Calcium channel blocking agents	Decrease total peripheral resistance without decreasing cardiac output	Heart failure may be aggravated; increased risk of digitalis toxicity; sodium and water retention do not occur.

◁ Table 4-21   Comparison of antihypertensive agents—cont'd

Classification	Effect	Comment
Vasodilators	Decrease peripheral resistance	Sympathetic nervous system and the renin-angiotensin-aldosterone system can be stimulated; sodium and water retention can occur.
ACE inhibitors	Decrease peripheral resistance	Aldosterone release is inhibited; patients undergoing diuretic therapy may experience profound hypotension when ACE inhibitors are administered.

ACE, angiotensin converting enzyme.

◁ Table 4-22   Sympatholytic agents

Drug		Usual Dosage
Alpha Adrenergic Blocking Agents		
Doxazosin mesylate (Cardura)	Oral	1 mg qd
Prazosin (Minipress)	Oral	1 mg bid-tid
	Range	6-15 mg qd
	Maximum	20 mg qd
Terazosin (Hytrin)	Oral	1 mg hs
	Range	1-5 mg qd
	Maximum	20 mg qd
Centrally Acting Agents		
Clonidine (Catapres)	Oral	0.1-0.8 mg in divided doses
	Maximum	1.2 mg qd
	Transdermal	1 patch/week (0.1-0.3 mg qd)

Continued.

Table 4-22   Sympatholytic agents—cont'd

Drug		Usual Dosage
Guanfacine (Tenex)	Oral	1 mg hs
Guanabenz (Wyten-sin)	Oral	4 mg bid initially
	Maximum	32 mg qd
Methyldopa (Aldo-met)	Oral	250 mg bid
	Maximum	2000 mg qd
	Infusion	500-1000 mg diluted in 100-200 ml D_5W q 6h

Description

Alpha adrenergic blocking agents block alpha 1 receptors, which are predominantly found in the vasculature, resulting in arterial and venous dilatation. Centrally acting agents stimulate alpha 2 receptors, which inhibit the release of norepinephrine. This action decreases sympathetic nervous system activity, which produces a hypotensive effect.

Clinical Alert

Concurrent use of alpha adrenergic blocking agents or centrally acting agents and other drugs that affect cardiovascular function may potentiate or antagonize the pharmacologic effects of these drugs.

Administration Precautions: Alpha Adrenergic Blocking Agents

- Use cautiously in patients with angina and renal impairment.
- Sodium and water retention may occur.
- Initial dosing may produce severe orthostatic hypotension for 30 minutes to 2 hours afterward. Caution patients to rise slowly from a supine position.
- Administer medication at bedtime to avoid the "first-dose orthostatic hypotensive reaction" described above.
- Do not administer if patient is experiencing symptomatic hypotension.

Patient Assessment: Alpha Adrenergic Blocking Agents

- Evaluate blood pressure control.
- Check weight daily for possible fluid retention.
- See Reportable Adverse Effects, which follow.

Reportable Adverse Effects: Alpha Adrenergic Blocking Agents

- Symptomatic hypotension; systolic blood pressure <90 mm Hg, dizziness, and fainting.
- Chest pain, palpitations, and dysrhythmias.
- Signs and symptoms of rebound hypertension: tachycardia, restlessness, and sweating.
- Fluid retention (increase in weight or edema).

Administration Precautions: Centrally Acting Agents

- Use cautiously in patients with coronary insufficiency.
- These agents can produce orthostatic hypotension.
- Do not administer if patient is experiencing symptomatic hypotension.
- Rebound hypertension can occur if these agents are abruptly discontinued.
- Sedation and drowsiness can occur; take at bedtime to decrease daytime drowsiness.
- Dental caries and periodontal disease can develop when using these agents.

Patient Assessment: Centrally Acting Agents

- Evaluate blood pressure control.
- Check for fluid retention (increase in weight or edema).
- See Reportable Adverse Effects, which follow.

Reportable Adverse Effects: Centrally Acting Agents

- Symptomatic hypotension; systolic blood pressure <90 mm Hg, dizziness, and fainting.
- Chest pain, palpitations, dysrhythmias, weakness, and shortness of breath.
- Signs and symptoms of rebound hypertension: tachycardia, restlessness, and sweating.
- Fluid retention.
- CNS changes, including mental depression, confusion, and irritability.

Administration Precautions: Specific Agents

Methyldopa

- Can produce autoimmune effects.
- Do not administer to patients with active liver disease.
- Parkinson's disease may be exacerbated.

- Hemolytic anemia may develop.
- Tolerance may develop.
- IV methyldopa should be administered over a period of 30 to 60 minutes.

Clonidine

- Transdermal units should not be cut or trimmed; avoid areas of skin irritation, scarring, and calluses.

Reportable Adverse Effects: Specific Agents

Methyldopa

- Fever, sore throat, hepatitis, bleeding, leukopenia, granulocytopenia, and thrombocytopenia.

Beta Adrenergic Blocking Agents

See discussion of these agents on p. 166.

Calcium Channel Blocking Agents

See p. 174 for a discussion of these agents.

Diuretic Agents

See discussion of these agents on p. 196.

Vasodilator Agents

Vasodilator agents are listed in Table 4-23.

Description

These agents reduce blood pressure by directly relaxing arteriolar smooth muscle, which results in dilatation of the vessel and a reduction in peripheral resistance. Sodium nitroprusside and minoxidil relax both arteriolar and venous smooth muscle and are referred to as balanced vasodilators. Sodium nitroprusside is the drug of choice for treating hypertensive crisis. It is given only intravenously and has a rapid onset and brief half-life.

Clinical Alert

Concurrent use of vasodilators and other drugs that affect cardiovascular function can potentiate or antagonize the pharmacologic effects of these drugs.

X, Table 4-23 Vasodilator agents

Drug		Usual Dosage
Diazoxide (Hyperstat)	IV	1-3 mg/kg; repeat in 5-15 min if necessary
Hydralazine (Apresoline)	Oral	25 mg bid
	Maximum	300 mg/day
	IV	10-40 mg; repeat as necessary
Minoxidil (Loniten)	Oral	5 mg/day initially
	Maintenance	10-40 mg/day
	Maximum	100 mg/day
Sodium nitroprusside (Nipride)	Infusion	50 mg/500 ml D_5W; (1 ml = 100 μg) at 0.1-5.0 μg/kg/min
	Maximum	10 μg/kg/min

Administration Precautions: Vasodilator Agents

- Use cautiously in patients with coronary insufficiency, because myocardial oxygen consumption can be increased (increase in heart rate and contractility secondary to decreased BP).
- Monitor blood pressure every 5 minutes during the intravenous administration of vasodilators.
- Orthostatic hypotension can occur.
- Fluid retention can occur.

Patient Assessment: Vasodilator Agents

- Evaluate blood pressure control.
- See Reportable Adverse Effects, which follow.

Reportable Adverse Effects: Vasodilator Agents

- Symptomatic hypotension: systolic blood pressure <90 mm Hg, dizziness, and fainting.
- Chest pain, dysrhythmias.
- Fluid retention (weight gain and ankle edema).
- Rebound hypertension.

Administration Precautions: Specific Agents

Diazoxide

- Use cautiously in diabetic patients since hypoglycemic medi-

cation may need adjusting; check blood sugar level.
- Administer through a peripheral line to prevent cardiac dysrhythmias.
- Administer undiluted over a 30-second period; a longer infusion time will decrease effectiveness.
- Monitor blood pressure every 5 to 15 minutes until stabilized.

Hydralazine

- Contraindicated in mitral valvular rheumatic heart disease because pulmonary artery pressures may increase.
- Systemic lupus erythematosus may develop when high doses are administered.

Minoxidil

- Pericardial effusion can occur.
- Excess hair growth usually develops 3 to 6 weeks after beginning therapy.
- Use cautiously in patients with pheochromocytoma, since increased catecholamine release can occur.

Nitroprusside

- Use cautiously in patients with hepatic impairment, renal impairment, or hypothyroidism.
- Arterial monitoring is recommended during infusion; if a rapid fall in blood pressure occurs, stop the infusion, put the patient in a supine position, and elevate the legs.
- Use an infusion control device to regulate the dosage.
- Do not exceed 10 μg/kg/minute.
- Tolerance may occur, which may be the first sign of toxicity.
- Risk of cyanide toxicity increases if the drug is infused longer than 72 hours or in patients with renal or hepatic impairment.
- Protect agent from light during administration; the solution normally has a brownish tint.

Reportable Adverse Effects: Specific Agents

Diazoxide

- Elevated blood glucose levels.

Hydralazine

- Blood dyscrasias, sore throat, fever, joint pain, and increase in ANA titer.
- Anxiety, flushing, numbness, and paresthesia.

Minoxidil

- Flushing, paresthesia, and shortness of breath.

Nitroprusside

- Toxic effects: excessive sweating, muscle twitching, nervousness and anxiety, blurred vision, delirium, headache, nausea and vomiting, ringing in the ears, and shortness of breath.
- Elevated serum cyanide or thiocyanate levels (see Appendix F).

Angiotensin-Converting Enzyme Inhibitors

Angiotensin-converting enzyme inhibitors are listed in Table 4-24.

Description

Angiotensin-converting enzyme (ACE) inhibitors reduce blood pressure by interfering with the renin-angiotensin-aldosterone system. By blocking the conversion of angiotensin I to the potent vasoconstrictor angiotensin II (see Figures 4-2 and 4-4) and inhibiting aldosterone release (aldosterone stimulation results in sodium and water retention, which increases intravascular volume and BP), peripheral arterial resistance is reduced. ACE inhibitors also break down bradykinin (a potent vasodilator) and inhibit sympathetic nervous system pressor response. Captopril and enalapril have been shown to reduce the incidence of overt heart failure and improve survival in patients with asymptomatic left ventricular dysfunction.

Clinical Alert

Concurrent use of ACE inhibitors and other drugs that affect cardiovascular function can potentiate or antagonize the pharmacologic effects of these drugs.

Administration Precautions: ACE Inhibitors

- Use these agents cautiously in patients with renal impairment, coronary artery disease, hyperkalemia, and recent MI.
- Patients currently taking diuretics may experience an excessive drop in blood pressure when ACE inhibitors are initiated.
- Severe hypotension can occur in patients who are sodium and volume depleted (i.e., patients with congestive heart failure).
- Do not administer if systolic blood pressure is <90 mm Hg, or if patient is dizzy or faint.

Table 4-24 **Angiotensin-converting enzyme inhibitors**

Drug	Indication and Usual Dosage	
Benazepril (Lotensin)	High blood pressure:	
	Oral	10 mg qd
	Maintenance	20-40 mg qd
Captopril (Capoten)	High blood pressure:	
	Oral	12.5-25 mg bid-tid
	Maximum	300-450 mg qd
	Heart failure:	
	Oral	12.5-25 mg tid
	Range	25-100 mg bid-tid
Enalapril maleate (Vasotec)	High blood pressure:	
	Oral	2.5-5 mg qd
	Range	10-40 mg qd
	IV	1.25 mg q6h; administer over 5 min
	Heart failure:	
	Oral	2.5 mg qd-bid
	Maintenance	5-20 mg qd
	Maximum	Up to 40 mg qd
Fosinopril (Monopril)	High blood pressure:	
	Oral	10 mg qd
	Maintenance	20-40 mg qd
Lisinopril (Zestril, Prinivil)	High blood pressure:	
	Oral	10 mg qd
	Range	20-40 mg qd
Quinapril (Accupril)	High blood pressure:	
	Oral	10 mg qd
	Maintenance	20-80 mg qd
Ramipril (Altace)	High blood pressure:	
	Oral	2.5 mg qd
	Maintenance	2.5-20 mg qd

- Renal perfusion may decrease with use of ACE inhibitors.
- Patients taking potassium supplements may develop hyperkalemia.
- Neutropenia or agranulocytosis can develop in patients with autoimmune diseases.
- Skin reactions can occur and require dosage reduction, withdrawal, or use of an antihistamine.
- Administer ACE inhibitors 1 hour before meals, since absorption is affected when taken with food.

Patient Assessment: ACE Inhibitors

- Evaluate blood pressure control.
- See Reportable Adverse Effects, which follow.

Reportable Adverse Effects: ACE Inhibitors

- Symptomatic hypotension: systolic blood pressure <90 mm Hg, dizziness, or fainting.
- Chest pain and shortness of breath.
- Blood dyscrasias: neutropenia and agranulocytosis
- Fever, chills, sore throat, and mouth sores.
- Skin rash, joint pain, persistent cough.
- Elevated serum potassium, BUN, and creatinine.
- Signs of hyperkalemia (see Table 4-18).

Antihyperlipidemic Agents

Overview

Elevated serum cholesterol levels increase the risk for cardiovascular disorders and have a major impact on morbidity and mortality. Elevated high-density lipoprotein levels, however, are associated with a decreased risk of coronary artery disease. Hyperlipidemic disorders can be genetic; secondary to such disorders as obesity, diabetes, or alcoholism; or produced by certain drugs (Table 4-25). Antihyperlipidemic agents (Table 4-26) interfere with the normal metabolism of cholesterol, triglycerides, and lipoproteins to reduce serum lipid levels. Lipid-lowering drugs are selected for their effect on specific lipoprotein disorders and are prescribed when dietary changes fail to work.

Description

Antihyperlipidemic agents affect either the production, catabolism, or removal of lipoproteins. Clofibrate and gemfibrozil lower triglyceride levels. Gemfibrozil increases HDL cholesterol. HMG CoA reductase inhibitors impair cholesterol synthesis and increase LDL receptor activity in the liver, which aids in the removal of LDL. Lovastatin is currently the most effective drug used to lower LDL cholesterol levels; pravastatin and simvastatin have similar effects. Bile acid sequestrants aid the removal of LDL by increasing LDL receptor activity. Niacin interferes with the synthesis and release of very low-density lipoproteins (VLDL) by the liver. Niacin lowers triglycerides and LDL cholesterol and increases HDL cho-

Table 4-25   **Drugs that affect lipid levels**

Drug Classification	Effect on Lipid Levels
Alpha adrenergic blockers	↓ LDL ↑ HDL
Beta blockers without ISA	↑ Triglycerides ↓ HDL
Calcium channel blockers	0/↓ LDL 0/↑ HDL
Diuretics*	↑ Triglycerides
Estrogens	↑ Triglycerides
Oral contraceptives	↑ Triglycerides
Progestins	↑ Cholesterol

*Indapamide has no effect on lipoproteins. HDL, High-density lipoproteins. LDL, Low-density lipoproteins. ↑, increase. ↓, decrease. 0, no change.

Table 4-26   **Antihyperlipidemic agents**

Drug		Usual Dosage
Fibric Acid Derivatives		
Clofibrate (Atromid-S)	Oral	1 g bid
Gemfibrozil (Lopid)	Oral	600 mg bid
	Range	900-1500 mg qd
Hydroxymethylglutaryl Coenzyme A (HMG CoA) Reductase Inhibitors		
Lovastatin (Mevacor)	Oral	20 mg qd
	Range	20-80 mg qd
	Maximum	80 mg qd
Pravastatin (Pravachol)	Oral	10-20 mg qd
Simvastatin (Zocor)	Oral	5-10 mg qd
Bile Acid Sequestrants		
Cholestyramine (Questran)	Oral	8-16 g bid
	Maximum	24 g/day
Colestipol (Colestid)	Oral	5-10 g tid
Other		
Niacin	Oral	1 g tid
	Range	3-6 g/day
Probucol (Lorelco)	Oral	250-500 mg bid
	Maximum	500 mg bid

lesterol. Probucol reduces LDL and HDL cholesterol levels. Side effects of antihyperlipidemic agents are mainly experienced in the gastrointestinal tract. However, clofibrate may cause dysrhythmias and probucal may prolong the QT interval.

Administration Precautions: Specific Agents

Fibric acid derivatives

- Avoid in patients with primary biliary cirrhosis.
- May increase risk of death from noncardiac causes.
- Risk for cholelithiasis is increased.

HMG CoA reductase inhibitors

- Long-term safety has not been established.
- Liver transaminase levels may be affected.
- Patient's eyes should be checked regularly for formation of lens opacities.

Bile acid sequestrants

- Accidental inhalation of powder or granules may occur. Instruct patients to mix the drug completely after allowing it to sit in approximately 150 ml of liquid for 2 minutes.
- Contraindicated in severe constipation: fecal impaction may occur.
- Interferes with other medications; take medications 1 hour before or 4 hours after the bile acid sequestrant.

Niacin

- Do not give to patients with peptic ulcer disease, liver disease, hyperuricemia, or gout.
- Patients develop a tolerance to flushing, but flushing tendency returns if dosage is interrupted. Ingesting niacin on an empty stomach may help reduce flushing. Premedication with aspirin or a nonsteroidal antiinflammatory agent may also help reduce flushing.

Probucol

- Women should wait at least 6 months after terminating probucol therapy to become pregnant.
- This drug should not be used in patients with primary biliary cirrhosis.

- Exercise caution in administering this drug to cardiac patients.
- Avoid using this drug in patients taking drugs that can prolong the QT interval.

Patient Assessment: Antihyperlipidemic Agents

- Evaluate serum lipid levels.
- See Reportable Adverse Effects, which follow.

Reportable Adverse Effects: Specific Agents

Fibric acid derivatives

- Abnormal blood counts, liver function tests, and lipid levels.

HMG CoA reductase inhibitors

- Elevated liver function tests.
- Cataract development.

Bile acid sequestrants

- Constipation and fecal impaction.

Niacin

- Abnormal liver function tests, serum glucose and uric acid levels.

Probucol

- Prolongation of the QT interval, dysrhythmias.

Hematologic Agents

Overview

A number of pharmacologic agents affect hemostasis and are clinically useful in preventing blood clot formation, dissolving formed clots, and reducing the risk for arterial thromboembolism. Some cardiovascular conditions that favor thrombosis include atrial fibrillation, valvular disease, prosthetic valves, angina, acute Q wave myocardial infarction, and coronary artery bypass graft surgery.

Normally, hemostasis is achieved through platelet aggregation/adhesion and activation of the cascade of coagulation factors. Although two pathways of clot formation exist, the end result is thrombin production and the transformation of fibrinogen to fibrin (Figure 4-5). A fibrinolytic mechanism that balances the hemostasis process removes or lyses clots. This mechanism prevents excessive

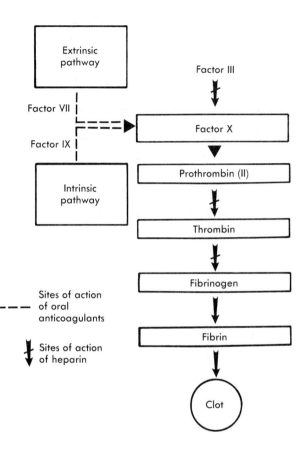

Figure 4-5
Coagulation cascade and sites of action of anticoagulant agents. The clotting process is activated by an extrinsic and an intrinsic pathway. Factor X is activated by factors IX, XI, and XII and kallikrein of the intrinsic pathway and factors III, VII, XI, and XII and kallikrein of the extrinsic pathway. Oral anti-coagulants interfere with vitamin K, which is responsible for formation of factors II, VII, IX, and X. Heparin reduces the amount of factor III (thromboplastin) and slows thrombin formation and the conversion of fibrinogen to fibrin.

intravascular clotting. Plasmin and plasminogen (inactive form of plasmin) are the enzymes involved in degrading and dissolving clots. Plasmin digests fibrin and fibrinogen, which produces fibrin split products.

Anticoagulant, thrombolytic, and antiplatelet agents interfere with the body's hemostatic functioning to prevent or alleviate obstruction to blood flow. Major side effects include bleeding, hemorrhagic necrosis, adrenal hemorrhages, and thrombocytopenia.

Anticoagulant Agents

Table 4-27 lists anticoagulant agents.

Description

Heparin, a parenteral anticoagulant, impairs the coagulation process (see Figure 4-5) at several sites in both the intrinsic and extrinsic clotting systems to inhibit thrombin formation and inactivate thrombin. It is not a fibrinolytic but prevents stabilization of a fibrin clot. Large doses of heparin are necessary to inactivate thrombin, in comparison to the dosage required to inhibit thrombin formation. In addition to heparin's therapeutic use in clinical conditions, it is used with specialized equipment (dialysis and cardiopulmonary bypass machines) and therapies (PTCA).

Coumarin derivatives (dicumarol, warfarin) are oral anticoagulants that inhibit vitamin K synthesis and thus prevent the formation of vitamin K–dependent procoagulation factors in the liver.

When an immediate anticoagulant effect is needed, heparin is the best choice. Its onset is immediate with the intravenous route, and it has a half-life of 1 to 6 hours. Coumarin derivatives are used

Table 4-27   Anticoagulant agents

Drug		Usual Dosage*
Heparin	Low dose	Subcutaneous 5000 U q 8-12h
	Therapeutic	IV, 10,000 U initially; 5000-10,000 U q 4-6h
	Infusion	1000 U/hr
Warfarin	Oral	10-15 mg qd, initially
	Maintenance	2-10 mg qd

*Dosages are adjusted according to coagulation test results.

for long-term anticoagulation. When switching the patient from heparin to an oral anticoagulant, both agents are generally administered concurrently until the desired prothrombin time is achieved.

Clinical Alert

Concurrent administration of several drugs or diet changes can alter the effectiveness of anticoagulants.

Administration Precautions: Anticoagulant Agents

- Anticoagulants are contraindicated in patients with active bleeding, recent surgery, hemophilia, pericarditis, or uncontrolled hypertension.
- Exercise caution when administering to patients with liver impairment.
- Effectiveness of anticoagulants can be altered when other medications are added or removed from the patient's regimen.
- Avoid intramuscular injections and invasive procedures in patients receiving anticoagulants.
- The antidote for coumadin is vitamin K; protamine sulfate is the antidote for heparin.
- The activated partial thromboplastin time (APTT) or partial thromboplastin time (PTT) for heparin therapy is usually 1.5 to 2.5 × the control; prothrombin time (PT) for coumadin therapy is usually 1.2 to 1.5 × the control, or an INR (international normalized ratio) of 2.0 to 3.0.
- Heparin can prolong PT when given by single IV injection; draw blood for PT just before the single IV dose.
- Clotting studies are usually not monitored with low-dose therapy, since the risk of bleeding is minimal.

Patient Assessment: Anticoagulant Agents

- Evaluate APTT/PTT for patients on heparin therapy.
- Evaluate PT or INR for patients on oral anticoagulant therapy.
- See Reportable Adverse Effects, which follow.

Reportable Adverse Effects: Anticoagulant Agents

- Notify physician if coagulation studies are not within the therapeutic range.
- Signs of covert (abdominal pain, joint or back pain) and overt bleeding.
- Thrombocytopenia (a mild form can occur 2 to 4 days into

therapy; a serious form of thrombocytopenia that can lead to thrombolic complications and organ infarction may occur after the eighth day of therapy).

Thrombolytic Agents

Thrombolytic agents are listed in Table 4-28.

Description

Thrombolytic agents lyse thrombi by converting plasminogen to plasmin (an enzyme that degrades fibrin clots, fibrinogen, and other clotting factors) to restore blood flow through the occluded vessel. Therapy with thrombolytic agents in the treatment of coronary thrombosis is aimed at reducing or limiting the size of the infarct by dissolving thrombi. As blood flow is restored, reperfusion dysrhythmias may occur. Other thromboembolic disorders, such as deep vein thrombosis and pulmonary embolus, may also be treated with these agents.

Thrombolytic agents are clot- or non-clot-specific. A comparison of thrombolytic agents can be found in Table 4-29. Non-clot-specific agents create a systemic thrombolytic state that presents a great risk of bleeding to the patient. A tissue plasminogen activator (t-PA) is a fibrinolytic agent and remains relatively inactive until it comes in contact with a thrombus and binds to fibrin. Fibrinolytic agents are less likely to contribute to systemic bleeding because they are clot-specific. Alteplase (sometimes referred to as t-PA) has the property of binding to fibrin to convert plasminogen to plasmin, thereby minimizing a systemic lytic state (Figure 4-6).

Clinical Alert

Thrombolytic Therapy is discussed on p. 241.

Administration Precautions: Thrombolytic Agents

- Contraindications include: active bleeding, recent surgery, hemorrhagic stroke, prolonged or traumatic CPR, recent intracranial or intraspinal surgery or trauma, tendencies toward bleeding, uncontrolled high blood pressure, suspected aortic dissection, or intracranial disorders.
- Bleeding is a major problem with thrombolytic agents.
- Be prepared to stop the infusion and administer blood prod-

X Table 4-28   Thrombolytic agents

Drug	Indication and Usual Dosage*	
Circulating Plasminogen Activators		
Antistreplase (Eminase)	Acute myocardial infarction:	
	IV	30 units over 2 to 5 min
Streptokinase (Streptase)	Acute myocardial infarction:	
	Intracoronary	20,000 IU initially, then 2000 IU/min over 60 min
	IV	1,500,000 IU over 1 hour
	Venous thromboembolism:	
		250,000 IU over 30 min
	Maintenance	100,000 IU/hr for 72 hr
Urokinase (Abbokinase)	Acute myocardial infarction:	
	Intracoronary	6000 IU/min
	IV	2,000,000-3,000,000 IU over 30 min
	Venous thromboembolism:	
		4000 IU/kg rapid infusion; 4000 IU/kg/hr for 24 hr
Tissue Plasminogen Activator		
Alteplase (Activase)	Acute myocardial infarction:	
	Initially 6-10 mg IV over 1-2 min, then a lytic dose of 50-54 mg the first hour	
	Maintenance: 20 mg the 2nd hour, 20 mg the 3rd hour, for a total of 100 mg	
	For patients <65 kg: A total dose of 1.25 mg/kg; bolus and first hour dose should equal three fifths of the total dose; second and third hour dosing should each equal one fifth of the total dose.	
	Pulmonary embolism:	
	IV	100 mg over 2 hr

*Clinical studies continue to investigate optimal dosage.

Table 4-29   Comparison of thrombolytic agents

Agent	Clot Specific	Systemic Effect	Antigenic Effect	Half-life
Alteplase	Y	minimal	N	5-8 min
Antistreplase	N	Y	Y	120 min
SK	N	Y	Y	18 min
UK	N	Y	N	20 min

SK, Streptokinase, UK, urokinase, Y, yes. N, no.

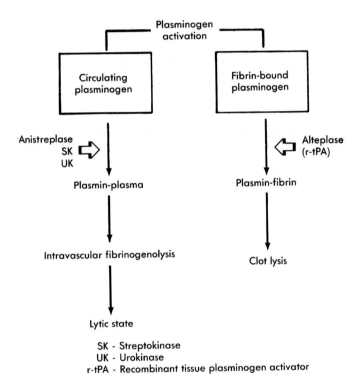

Figure 4-6
Action sites of thrombolytic agents. Activation of plasmino-gen produces a clot lysing process. Thrombolytic agents act as plasminogen activators and have either an affinity for cir-culating (plasma) plasminogen (nonclot specific) or fibrin-bound plasminogen (clot specific).

ucts. Avoid administering dextrans because they exhibit antiplatelet activity. Aminocaproic acid, which inhibits plasminogen activator substances, may be ordered.

- Concurrent administration of antiplatelet and anticoagulant agents to patients receiving thrombolytic agents is not recommended.

Patient Assessment: Thrombolytic Agents

- Evaluate resolution of chest discomfort, normalization of ST segment, and onset of reperfusion dysrhythmias (see section on Thrombolytic Therapy, p. 241).
- See Reportable Adverse Effects, which follow.

Reportable Adverse Effects: Thrombolytic Agents

- Signs of overt or covert bleeding.
- Onset of chest discomfort, ST segment elevation, or dysrhythmias.

Administration Precautions: Specific Agents
Streptokinase and Antistreplase

- Patients receiving repeated doses of SK may experience an allergic reaction; premedication with a nonsteroidal antiinflammatory agent may be used.
- Severe hypotension can occur.

Reportable Adverse Effects: Specific Agents
Streptokinase and Antistreplase

- Allergic reaction.
- Hypotension.

Antiplatelet Agents

Antiplatelet agents are listed in Table 4-30.

Description

Platelets play a role in the development of cardiovascular disorders, including coronary artery thrombosis. Antiplatelet agents interfere with platelet function by reducing platelets' ability to aggregate and are used primarily to reduce the risk of thromboembolic events in patients with prosthetic cardiac valves. These agents are

Table 4-30   Antiplatelet agents

Drug		Usual Dosage
Aspirin	Oral	20-325 mg qd
Dipyridamole (Persantine)	Oral	75-100 mg tid-qid
	Infusion	250 mg/250 ml D_5W; (1 ml = 1 mg) at 10 mg/hr
Sulfinpyrazone (Anturane)	Oral	100-200 mg bid

also used to decrease myocardial reinfarction and prolong the patency of coronary artery bypass grafts.

Sulfinpyrazone and aspirin inhibit the enzyme (cyclooxygenase) reaction that results in thromboxane A_2, which is a potent vasoconstrictor and platelet-aggregating–stimulating substance. Dipyridamole inhibits the platelet release reaction and platelet aggregation by inhibiting platelet phosphodiesterase. Major side effects include gastrointestinal upset and bleeding.

Administration Precautions: Antiplatelet Agents

- Concurrent use of anticoagulant or thrombolytic agents with antiplatelet agents increases the risk for bleeding.
- Concurrent use of ulcerogenic drugs increases the risk of GI bleeding.
- Patients with active bleeding or hemophilia should not receive these agents.
- Avoid administering antiplatelet agents to patients with thrombocytopenia.

Administration Precautions: Specific Agents

Aspirin

- Administer with a full glass of water and have patient sit upright for 15 to 30 minutes afterward.
- Allow a 1- to 2-hour interval between enteric-coated aspirin and antacids or H_2 antagonists (cimetidine or ranitidine).
- GI bleeding may occur.

Dipyridamole

- Exercise caution when administering to patients with hypotension.
- Chest pain may occur (coronary steal phenomenon).

Sulfinpyrazone

· Avoid administering to patients with renal stones.

Patient Assessment: Antiplatelet Agents

· Evaluate bleeding time and platelet aggregation test.
· See Reportable Adverse Effects, which follow.

Reportable Adverse Effects: Specific Agents

Aspirin

· Loss of hearing, ringing or buzzing in the ears, severe diarrhea, severe or continuous headache, severe drowsiness, fast and deep breathing.
· Signs of overt or covert bleeding.

Dipyridamole

· Chest pain.
· Signs of overt or covert bleeding.

Sulfinpyrazone

· Renal impairment.
· Convulsions, persistent nausea and vomiting, severe stomach pain, clumsiness or unsteadiness.
· Signs of overt or covert bleeding.

Peripheral Vascular Agents

Overview

Atherosclerosis of the arterial system is the leading cause of arterial insufficiency. Obstruction of arterial blood flow either by vasospasm or atherosclerosis impairs adequate delivery of oxygen and nutrients to the tissues, which can cause the patient pain and discomfort. Peripheral vascular agents are used to improve circulation and provide symptomatic relief for both vasospastic and atherosclerotic occlusive disease. These agents include vasodilators, beta adrenergic stimulants, hemorrheologic agents, and calcium channel blocking agents. The usefulness of vasodilators and beta adrenergic stimulants is controversial, however, the hemorrheologic agent has been shown to improve perfusion and relieve symptoms. Calcium channel blockers (nifedipine in particular) have been used in vasospastic disease and have demonstrated symptomatic benefits. Calcium channel blocking agents are discussed on p. 174. Major cardiovascular side effects include hypotension, dysrhythmias, palpitations, and chest pain. These agents, with the exception of pentoxifylline (Trental), have a greater vasodilator effect on peripheral vessels than on coronary or cerebral vessels; therefore, they may further decrease blood flow to ischemic areas and thus are responsible for a possible "steal effect."

Peripheral Vascular Agents

Peripheral vascular agents are listed in Table 4-31.

Description

Isoxsuprine and nylidrin increase blood flow to distal tissues by vasodilating blood vessels. Nylidrin stimulates beta 2 receptors, causing skeletal arteries and arterioles to dilate; isoxsuprine dilates vascular smooth muscle walls directly. In addition, isoxsuprine is a cardiac stimulant. Pentoxifylline, on the other hand, is an agent that improves oxygen supply to tissues by increasing the flexibility of red blood cells and lowering blood viscosity.

Calcium Channel Blocking Agents

See p. 174 for a discussion of these agents.

Administration Precautions: Specific Agents

Hemorrheologic agent

- Do not administer to patients who are allergic to xanthines (caffeine or theophylline), since this agent is a methylxanthine derivative.
- Exercise caution when administering to patients with coronary

Table 4-31   **Peripheral vascular agents**

Drug		Usual Dosage
Hemorrheologic Agent		
Pentoxifylline (Trental)	Oral	400 mg tid
Beta Adrenergic Stimulating Agents		
Nylidrin (Arlidin)	Oral	3-12 mg tid-qid
Isoxsuprine (Vasodilan, Vaso-prine)	Oral	10-20 mg tid-qid

artery disease; they may be at increased risk for experiencing adverse effects.

Beta adrenergic stimulating agents

- Exercise caution when administering to patients with heart disease; a "steal effect" may be produced, resulting in coronary ischemia; increased heart rate may increase myocardial oxygen demand in patients with angina and recent MI.
- Peptic ulcer disease may be aggravated because gastric acid secretion is increased.

Patient Assessment: Peripheral Vascular Agents

- Evaluate pain and walking endurance.
- See Reportable Adverse Effects, which follow.

Reportable Adverse Effects: Specific Agents
Hemorrheologic agent

- Chest pain and dysrhythmias.
- Signs of overdose include drowsiness, flushing, faintness, unusual excitement, and seizures.

Beta adrenergic stimulating agents

- Hypertension, tachycardia, dysrhythmias.
- Signs of overdose: blurred vision, angina, metallic taste, fever, and inability to void.

Selected bibliography

American Heart Association: Guidelines for Cardiopulmonary Resuscitation and Emergency Cardiac Care, *JAMA* 268(16):2171-2250, 1992.

American Medical Association: *Drug evaluations,* Philadelphia, 1991, Saunders.

Drugs for cardiac arrhythmias *Medical letter,* 33(846):55-60, 1991.

Facts and comparisons, St Louis, 1993, Lippincott.

Gahart B: *Intravenous medications,* ed 8, St Louis, 1992, Mosby.

Monrad, E: Thrombolysis: the need for a critical review, *Journal of the American College of Cardiology* 18(6):1573-1578, 1991.

Position paper, national education programs working group report on the management of patients with hypertension and high blood cholesterol, *Annals of Internal Medicine* 114(3):224-237, 1991.

Textbook of advanced cardiac life support, Dallas, 1990, American Heart Association.

United States Pharmacopeial Convention, Inc: *USPDI: drug information for the health care professional,* ed 12, Rockville, Maryland, 1992.

Select
Cardiovascular
Therapies

5

Cardiac Surgery

Description

Cardiac surgery is the treatment of choice for many forms of cardiac disease. The cardiopulmonary bypass machine facilitated the development and refinement of surgical techniques that have contributed to a decline in morbidity and mortality rates. Other advances, such as modifications in cardioplegia, which enhances myocardial preservation, and improved methods for hemodynamic monitoring have also had a positive impact on surgical results. Examples of cardiac surgery are listed in Table 5-1.

Cardiopulmonary (CP) bypass is used for major cardiac surgical procedures. The CP bypass machine oxygenates and pumps the patient's blood during the operation. As a result, it is not necessary for the patient's own heart and lungs to function, allowing for a quiet, relatively bloodless operative field for the surgeon. Concepts integral to CP bypass include hemodilution, anticoagulation, and hypothermia. Diluting the patient's blood (hemodilution) decreases its viscosity, enhancing flow and decreasing the risk of clotting. Hemodilution also decreases damage to the red blood cells, resulting in less hemolysis. Anticoagulation therapy is necessary to minimize clot formation as blood flows through the CP bypass machine. Hypothermia—cooling of the blood and, in turn, of the core body temperature—decreases metabolic demands while the patient is on CP bypass.

Myocardial preservation to prevent muscle damage is a major objective during cardiac surgery. The myocardium is protected via cold cardioplegic solution or topical iced saline. Hypothermia de-

☆ Table 5-1   **Examples of cardiac surgery**

Indication	Examples of Procedures
Coronary artery disease	Endarterectomy, coronary artery bypass, aneursymectomy
Valvular disease	Balloon valvuloplasty, commissurotomy, valve replacement
Congenital defects	Repair of ASD, VSD, coarctation, valve repair or replacement
Cardiovascular trauma	Repair of vessels or cardiac defect, pacemaker implantation
Cardiac tumor	Resection of tumor
Severe ventricular dysfunction	Insertion of ventricular assist device, heart transplantation, total artificial heart

creases myocardial oxygen consumption, and the cardioplegic solution causes sudden cessation of cardiac activity while also providing a supply of nutrients necessary for cardiac metabolism. The effects of normothermic blood cardioplegia (warm open heart surgery) are being investigated by some cardiovascular surgeons.

Complications

Complications of cardiac surgery (Table 5-2) are typically associated with preexisting medical problems, extended time on CP bypass, or procedural problems. They include perioperative myocardial infarction, hemorrhage, cardiac tamponade (see p. 234), dysrhythmias, hypotension, hypertension, fluid/electrolyte and acid/base imbalances, renal failure, respiratory failure, infection, and cerebrovascular accident.

Preoperative Care

Patient and family anxiety can be reduced with individualized preoperative teaching. See p. 235.

Postoperative Care

A major postoperative priority is the prevention of complications or, if that is not possible, early identification of complications so
Text continued on page 234.

Table 5-2   Complications of cardiac surgery

Complication	Possible Causes
Cardiovascular	
Decreased cardiac output	Hypovolemia, decreased contractility, PEEP
Hemorrhage	Surgical bleeder, inadequate heparin reversal, coagulopathy
Cardiac tamponade	Inadequate drainage from mediastinal tube
Myocardial infarction	Ineffective myocardial preservation during surgery, hypotension, hypertension, dysrhythmias, graft closure
Dysrhythmias	Preexisting heart disease, trauma of surgery, effects of cardiopulmonary bypass and hypothermia, electrolyte imbalance, acid/base imbalance, myocardial ischemia/infarction
Hypertension	Preexisting hypertension, fluid overload, delayed action of catecholamines stored in the capillaries during hypothermia, medication
Postpericardiotomy syndrome	Trauma to pericardium, immune response to pericardial injury
Pulmonary	
Atelectasis	Anesthetics, narcotics, effects of cardiopulmonary bypass (quiet lung, decreased surfactant, microemboli), pain, decreased mobility, interstitial edema
Hemothorax	Inadequate drainage from pleural chest tube
Pneumothorax	High tidal volumes and airway pressures of ventilator, incorrect placement of central line or endotracheal tube, entrance into pleural cavity at time of surgery

Table 5-2 Complications of cardiac surgery—cont'd

Complication	Possible Causes
Renal	
Decreased renal function	Effects of cardiopulmonary bypass (hemolysis, decreased renal perfusion, microemboli), hypovolemia, decreased ventricular function, vasopressor agents
Neurologic	
Altered level of consciousness	Sensory deprivation or overload, lack of sleep, unfamiliar environment, effects of cardiopulmonary bypass (microemboli, macroemboli, decreased cerebral perfusion), thrombus dislodged during surgery, air embolism, hypotension or hypertension, acid/base imbalance, some medications/anesthesia
Metabolic	
Fluid/electrolyte imbalance, acid/base imbalance	Stress response to trauma of surgery, effects of cardiopulmonary bypass (hemodilution, decreased tissue perfusion), loss of fluid, diuretics, blood transfusions
Infection	
Respiratory tract	Atelectasis, mechanical ventilation
Urinary tract	Urinary catheter
Incisional	Interruption of skin integrity due to surgery
Phlebitis	Intravenous lines
Valvular	Preexisting valve disease, valve prosthesis, surgical procedure, invasive lines
Sepsis	Invasive lines, debilitated state, poor nutrition

Cardiac Tamponade

Definition

Compression of the heart usually caused by blood/effusion in the pericardial sac, which increases intrapericardial pressure. This increased pressure impedes ventricular filling and, in turn, cardiac output.

Clinical Manifestations

Tachycardia
↑ CVP
Neck vein distention
Kussmaul's sign
Plateau pressure (equalization of right-sided and left-sided heart pressures)
↓ BP
Narrowed pulse pressure
Paradoxic pulse
Muffled or distant heart sounds
Decreased urinary output
Dyspnea, tachypnea
Anxiety, restlessness
Sudden decrease in amount of mediastinal tube drainage

Treatment

Pericardiocentesis (when mediastinal tube is not present)
Surgical removal of fluid or clot

BP, blood pressure. CVP, central venous pressure.

that appropriate intervention can be initiated. See Table 5-2 for complications of cardiac surgery. Accurate hemodynamic monitoring is especially important and must encompass recognition of the early indications of hypovolemia (e.g., paradoxic pressure curve and low or decreasing pulmonary artery wedge pressure) associated with the combined effects of rewarming and vasodilator therapy. Other areas of focus include assessment of fluid losses (especially monitor mediastinal tube drainage to detect hemorrhage or tamponade), evaluation of appropriate laboratory tests (hemoglobin, hematocrit, electrolyte, coagulation studies, and arterial blood gases),

Preoperative Teaching for the Patient Undergoing Cardiovascular Surgery

Teaching should be tailored to patient and family.
Topics to review may include:
  Surgical procedure
    Basic cardiovascular anatomy and physiology
    Brief pathophysiology related to specific problem (e.g., coronary artery disease, peripheral vascular disease)
    Patient understanding of procedure
    Location of incisions
  Preoperative routine
    Visits from surgeon, anesthesiologist, respiratory therapist, intensive care nurse
    Surgical prep, showers, shave
    Nothing by mouth
    Coughing and deep breathing instruction, use of spirometer
    Preoperative medications
  Operating room
    Insertion of invasive lines (arterial, intravenous)
    Holding area
    Patient understanding of anesthesia induction
  Postsurgical equipment and routines in the intensive care unit
    Endotracheal tube and ventilator
    Communication while intubated
    Lines and tubes (IVs, arterial line, mediastinal tubes, urinary catheter, pacing wires)
    Coughing and deep breathing
    Pain control
    Routine monitoring (continuous ECG, blood pressure, daily blood work, 12-lead ECG)
    Drinking and eating
    Ambulation
    Transfer from intensive care to nursing unit
  Orientation to intensive care unit
    Visiting hours
    Waiting area for family
    Method of communication with family
    Tour of unit if desired
  Additional patient and family questions

and titration of pharmacologic agents to maintain hemodynamic pressures within prescribed parameters. Careful patient assessment and evaluation of response to therapy allows any necessary changes to be made in a timely manner. Refer to Chapter 2 for additional information about patient assessment. Anxiety reduction is another postoperative concern. The patient and family should be included in up-to-date, caring communication and in decision making (when appropriate).

Peripheral Vascular Surgery

Description

Surgery may be the treatment of choice for some forms of peripheral vascular occlusive disease (PVOD). Refer to Chapter 1 for a discussion of PVOD. Arterial reconstructive procedures are palliative and are performed to improve tissue perfusion, relieve symptoms, and/or salvage limbs at risk for amputation. A variety of graft materials, including Dacron, Gortex, or saphenous vein(s), may be used to bypass blockages in peripheral vessels. Select surgical bypass procedures are described in Table 5-3.

Preoperative Care

Patient and family anxiety can be reduced with individualized preoperative teaching. See p. 235 for suggested topics.

Complications

The patient is at risk for hemorrhage, graft occlusion, and graft or wound infection following vascular surgery. Many patients with PVOD also have coronary artery disease, so perioperative or postoperative myocardial infarction is another potential complication.

Additional complications specific to aortofemoral bypass are intestinal ischemia/infarct (if blood supply to the bowel is interrupted) and prolonged ileus (because of manipulation of the bowel at the time of surgery). These complications do not occur with axillofemoral and femorofemoral bypass procedures because the abdominal cavity is not invaded. These procedures are therefore preferred for the high-risk patient. An additional benefit of femorofemoral bypass is that it can be performed under epidural or spinal anesthesia.

⚹ Table 5-3 **Select peripheral vascular surgical procedures**

Procedure	Description
Aortofemoral bypass	Graft from aorta to one or both common femoral arteries; bypasses blockage in terminal aorta and iliac arteries; incisions in abdomen and one or both groins
Femoropopliteal bypass	Graft from common femoral artery to popliteal artery above or below the knee; bypasses blockage in superficial femoral artery and popliteal artery; incisions in groin and above or below the knee
Femorotibial bypass	Graft from common femoral artery to anterior or posterior tibial artery; bypasses blockage in superficial femoral, popliteal, and tibial/peroneal arteries; incisions in groin and lower leg/ankle
Axillofemoral bypass	Graft from axillary artery tunneled subcutaneously and anastomosed to common femoral artery; bypasses blockage in aorta and iliac arteries; incisions in subclavicular area and groin; used for high-risk patients (e.g., those with concomitant pulmonary or cardiac disease or infection of an existing graft)
Femorofemoral bypass	Graft from one common femoral artery to the other femoral artery (donor artery must have no significant stenosis); bypasses iliac disease; incisions in both groins; used for high-risk patients (e.g., those with concomitant pulmonary or cardiac disease or infection of an existing graft)

A complication associated with below-the-knee bypass is compartment syndrome. Prolonged ischemia to the lower leg prior to revascularization may result in swelling of the calf muscles and subsequent compartment syndrome. As the muscles swell within the fascial compartment, increased pressure impairs blood flow to nerves and muscles. To relieve the increased pressure, emergency fasciotomy may be necessary.

Postoperative Care

Postoperative care focuses on maintaining graft patency, preventing wound and graft infection, and teaching the patient prudent health practices. Monitor both fluid status and blood pressure closely. Hypovolemia and/or hypotension may cause graft occlusion. Hypertension may cause bleeding.

Assess perfusion to the tissue by monitoring pulses, color, temperature, sensation, and movement of the affected extremity. Report any deterioration to the surgeon immediately. Signs and symptoms of compartment syndrome include change in motor function (i.e., loss of power or extreme pain with passive stretch) and severe pain at rest or pain not responding to analgesics. Distal pulses may persist until irreversible necrosis occurs.

Position the patient in such a manner as to avoid pressure on a subcutaneous graft (axillofemoral or femorofemoral), teach the patient to avoid kinking a graft (i.e., crossing legs, sharp hip flexion). Meticulous care of the wound site will help prevent infection. Notify the surgeon of elevated temperature, unusual wound tenderness, or purulent wound drainage. Patient education is imperative and should emphasize modification of risk factors and foot care. Chapter 6 discusses specific patient education information. If the patient has received a prosthetic graft, information about antibiotic prophylaxis before surgery or extensive dental work should also be provided.

Percutaneous Transluminal Coronary Angioplasty

Description

Percutaneous transluminal coronary angioplasty (PTCA) is a procedure developed to reestablish coronary artery blood flow to the myocardium. Stenotic coronary arteries are dilated via rapid balloon inflation and deflation that compresses atherosclerotic plaque against the arterial vessel wall. A patient willing to undergo percutaneous transluminal coronary angioplasty (PTCA) must be a candidate for coronary artery bypass graft (CABG) surgery, since abrupt occlusion of the coronary artery is a risk of PTCA. The ideal candidate has an isolated single-vessel lesion. However, patients with multivessel disease, unstable angina, acute myocardial infarction, stenosed grafts post-CABG, and post-thrombolytic therapy can benefit from PTCA.

The patient is taken to the catheterization laboratory, where a balloon-tipped catheter is inserted via femoral arteriotomy, advanced to the ostium of the coronary artery, and guided across the stenotic lesion. Heparin anticoagulation is initiated during the procedure. Predilatation pressure gradients are obtained. The balloon is then inflated and deflated quickly to compress the atherosclerotic lesion. Patients may receive nitroglycerin and calcium channel blocking agents during the procedure. The pressure gradient across the stenosis is measured postdilatation to determine the effects of the procedure. Several balloon inflations may be necessary to obtain successful dilatation or angioplasty. Successful angioplasty, according to the International Society and Federation of Cardiology and the World Health Organization,* includes a change in luminal diameter $\geq 20\%$ from pre-PTCA to post-PTCA, final diameter stenosis $< 50\%$ (if pre-PTCA diameter stenosis is $\geq 50\%$), and absence of major complications. Repeat angioplasty can be performed if restenosis occurs. Exercise testing and repeat angiograms are evaluated as part of the follow-up care.

Complications

The patient may experience chest pain or discomfort, vasovagal response, injury to the vessel with medial dissection, thrombus formation at the dilatation site, and bleeding or hematoma and thrombus formation at the puncture site. Major complications include death, MI, or the need for revascularization surgery.

Patient Preparation

Informed consent for PTCA and coronary artery bypass graft surgery should be obtained by the physician. Explanations about the

---

*Bourassa M. and others: Report of the joint ISFC/WHO task force on coronary angioplasty, Special Report, *Circulation,* 78(3):784, 1988.

procedure should include the need for NPO status; description of the catheterization laboratory, and patient expectations during the procedure (patient will be awake, may experience warm flushed feeling during contrast injection, and is immobilized during the procedure); and the postprocedural protocol (return to the intensive care unit, frequent monitoring of vital signs and assessment of peripheral circulation and the puncture site, bedrest with affected extremity kept straight, and elevation of the head of the bed [limited to a 30° angle]). The patient may resume meals post-PTCA, and activity may be resumed 4 to 6 hours after sheath removal. The patient is usually transferred out of the intensive care unit after 24 hours and discharged within 48 hours of the procedure.

Post-PTCA Care

Assess for bleeding, hematoma, or thrombus formation at the puncture site. Obtain frequent vital signs and check peripheral circulation of the involved extremity every 15 minutes the first hour; every 30 minutes the second hour, and hourly thereafter. Evaluate the patient's response to therapy; any evidence of restenosis (onset of chest pain or ST segment changes) should be reported immediately to the physician. Continuously monitor the patient for reperfusion dysrhythmias (bradycardia, heart block, ventricular tachycardia, or accelerated idioventricular rhythm).

Maintain patient on bedrest with the head of the bed elevated at a 30° angle or less, and immobilize the involved extremity. The patient may return from the catheterization laboratory with a heparin infusion, which is usually discontinued within 24 to 48 hours. Careful assessment for covert or overt bleeding and monitoring of PTT is critical in postangioplasty patients.

Removal of femoral sheaths usually occurs 4 to 6 hours after heparin cessation (if coagulation studies are normal). Apply direct pressure to the insertion site until hemostasis is achieved. Antiplatelet agents will be prescribed for the patient to prevent coronary artery restenosis. PTCA is not a cure for coronary artery disease. The patient should be educated about the disease, medications, risk factor modifications, signs and symptoms that need medical attention, and follow-up care.

Clinical Alert

Monitor patient closely for coronary artery restenosis (chest discomfort, ST segment changes, and dysrhythmias).

Thrombolytic Therapy

Description

Thrombolytic agents dissolve clots in acute MI so that blood flow to the myocardium can be reestablished and myocardial damage limited. Information on specific drugs can be found on p. 222. Early treatment can reduce infarct size, preserve left ventricular function, and decrease the incidence of congestive heart failure. Making an accurate diagnosis in potential candidates (Table 5-4) and assessing contraindications are critical to thrombolytic therapy. Contraindications include active bleeding, bleeding tendencies, recent surgery (<2 weeks) or significant trauma, uncontrolled high blood pressure (>200/120), hemorrhagic stroke, prolonged or traumatic CPR, suspected aortic dissection, pregnancy, intracranial disorders, and recent (<2 months) intracranial/intraspinal surgery or trauma.

Although successful reperfusion can be assessed angiographically, the presence of three noninvasive clinical parameters have been correlated with reperfusion. These markers—resolution of ischemic chest pain or discomfort, normalization of ST segments, and the appearance of dysrhythmias—are also characteristic of normal myocardial infarction evolution. However, these parameters may be useful as indicators of reperfusion if all three occur simultaneously.

Another indicator of successful reperfusion, although a late clinical marker, is the presence of an elevated cardiac enzyme and isoenzyme. Creatinine kinase (CK) and CK-MB peak earlier with a reperfused myocardium than with the natural evolution of acute MI. The peaks occur within 12 hours after the onset of symptoms

Table 5-4   Conventional inclusion criteria for thrombolytic therapy

Symptom	Chest pain or discomfort (ischemic pain) >30 minutes; unrelieved by nitroglycerin; <6 hours in duration
ECG changes	Consistent with acute MI: ST segment elevation in two contiguous leads (with ST segment depression in reciprocal leads); Q waves may or may not be present

in the reperfused myocardium, as opposed to 24 hours in the normally-evolving MI. This early peaking of CK and CK-MB is referred to as the CK "wash-out" phenomenon.

Complications

Bleeding is the major complication associated with thrombolytic therapy. Intracranial, internal, and surface bleeding can occur. Reperfusion dysrhythmias can also develop but do not require treatment unless cardiac output is compromised. Frequently observed dysrhythmias include accelerated idioventricular rhythm, ventricular tachycardia, bradycardia, and various forms of AV block. When accelerated idioventricular rhythm develops, cardiac output is not usually affected. However, it may decompensate to ventricular tachycardia (see Appendix H for treatment of ventricular tachycardia).

Reocclusion of the coronary artery, a life-threatening complication, requires immediate intervention. The first 24 hours following thrombolysis is critical, requiring early recognition of coronary artery reocclusion. Factors contributing to this complication include high-grade residual stenosis, coronary artery vasospasm, injury to the vessel, and residual thrombosis. Recurrent chest discomfort, ST segment elevation, and the appearance of dysrhythmias may indicate reocclusion of the coronary artery. Repeat thrombolysis, angioplasty, or revascularization may be required.

Patient Preparation

Obtain a patient history to identify any contraindications to therapy. Instruct the patient that venous access is required and bedrest with minimal movement is necessary. Inform the patient that scratching or self-inflicted injury can cause bleeding. Avoid subclavian or internal jugular venous access, since hemostasis is difficult to achieve at these sites.

Care During and After Thrombolytic Therapy

Evaluate the patient's response to thrombolytic therapy by monitoring for pain relief, normalization of ST segment, or reperfusion dysrhythmias. Treat dysrhythmias if the patient becomes hemodynamically unstable. Assess for covert or overt bleeding, check neurologic status every 2 hours, and monitor hemoglobin and hematocrit levels and coagulation studies. Test urine, feces, and emesis for occult blood; monitor IV sites for bleeding; assess for hematoma formation at arterial catheter site; monitor patient for retroperitoneal bleeding. Avoid injections and venipunctures if at all possible (use heparin or saline lock for drawing blood samples). Wait at least 24 hours after thrombolytic therapy before discontinuing IV sites.

Clinical Alert

Monitor the patient for reocclusion of the coronary artery (chest pain, ST segment changes, and dysrhythmias). Carefully observe the patient for bleeding.

Transplantation

Description

Heart transplantation is reserved for patients with end-stage heart disease. The transplant candidate usually has a life expectancy of less than 6 months and meets the NYHA class IV status. Most of the candidates are diagnosed with cardiomyopathy, congenital defect, ischemic heart disease, or valvular heart disease. Eisenmenger's complex and primary pulmonary hypertension are common indications for heart and lung transplantation.

Contraindications to heart transplantation include active infection, systemic disease, pulmonary hypertension, hepatic abnormalities, obesity, drug abuse, and mental illness.

Transplants can be heteroptic (leaving the native heart in place and "piggy-backing" the donor heart) or orthotopic (removing the diseased heart and replacing it with the donor heart). A third procedure combines heart and lung transplantation. The recipient's heart and lungs are removed as a unit and replaced with the donor organs.

Complications

Major post-transplantation problems include rejection, infection, complications of immunosuppressive therapy, and accelerated atherosclerosis.

Hyperacute rejection occurs within hours of surgery; acute rejection occurs after the fourth postoperative day; and chronic rejection, which is associated with a gradual loss of organ function, occurs over months. Immunosuppressive therapy is initiated to reduce the body's attempt to reject the transplanted organ(s) and must continue for the lifespan of the organ(s). Cyclosporine, prednisone, and azathioprine are currently used in immunosuppressive therapy. Acute rejection may be treated with corticosteroids, antithymocyte globulin, and OKT3.

Accelerated graft atherosclerosis in heart transplant recipients is a result of chronic rejection.

Infection is a major cause of death in heart transplant patients and is problematic immediately postoperatively and secondary to immunosuppressive drugs. Placing the patient in protective isolation is necessary to reduce the risk of infection.

In addition to infection, other adverse effects from immunosuppressive therapy include peptic ulcers, high blood pressure, organ dysfunction, pancreatitis, impaired healing, and steroid-induced diabetes. The use of cyclosporine has decreased morbidity and mortality resulting from infection. However, it can produce nephrotoxic effects.

Several diagnostic tests evaluate organ function, effects of pharmacologic agents, and the presence of infection or rejection, including ECGs; cardiac enzyme tests; complete blood counts; clotting studies; cultures of drainage, sputum, and blood; and endomyocardial biopsies. These tests are performed frequently during the postoperative period. Endomyocardial biopsies are currently used to confirm rejection but noninvasive diagnostic tests are under investigation.

Preoperative Care

The patient and family should be aware that surgery can occur at any hour and that a long wait for a donor heart may be necessary. Everyone involved should understand the risks of surgery and immunosuppressive therapy. An explanation of the thorough physical and psychosocial preoperative testing should be provided. Preoperative education concerning surgery and postoperative expectations are similar to that of any other open heart surgery.

Postoperative Care

Care of the transplant patient is similar to any other open heart surgical patient. However, protective isolation should be enforced. Patients are closely monitored for rejection, sepsis, and other adverse effects.

Follow-up care focuses on compliance with the medical regimen. Self-care instructions should include activity and dietary restrictions, administration of medication, signs and symptoms of infection and rejection, risk-factor modification; coughing and deep

breathing exercises, prevention of infection, and life-long follow-up care. The phone numbers of health team members and
other resources should be provided to facilitate the patient's adaptation to the transplant experience.

Other Therapies

Laser Therapy

A laser (light amplification by simulated emission of radiation)
emits energy at a specific wavelength and interacts with tissue to
produce various reactions, such as vaporization, coagulation, or hemostasis. These reactions depend on the type of laser used (CO_2,
Nd:YAG, and argon lasers are the most commonly used), the type
of tissue being irradiated, and the amount and duration of laser exposure. Laser therapy has been used on lesions in the brain, vocal
cords, cervix, skin, bronchus, bladder, and gastrointestinal tract.
The effects of laser therapy on calcified aortic valves, hypertrophic
cardiomyopathy, aberrant conduction pathways, and peripheral and
coronary artery atheroma are currently under investigation.

Although laser light has the ability to destroy atherosclerotic
plaque in both peripheral and coronary circulation, the technical aspects, effects on surrounding tissue, and long-term effects need further investigation. Cardiac perforation and tamponade have occurred as a result of technical difficulties in manipulating the laser.
Arterial walls have been damaged causing thrombosis and aneurysms. Embolization, reperfusion dysrhythmias, vasospasm, and
bleeding are other potential complications. Laser safety must be
ensured to protect the patient and health care team members.

Research is being conducted on various devices and delivery
systems (modification of fiberoptic tips, photodynamic therapy, and
excimer-pulsed laser angioplasty) to reduce the incidence of complications and determine optimal laser parameters in the treatment
of cardiovascular disease.

Intravascular Stents

A stent is an endoprosthesis, a pliable, self-expandable wire mesh
made from stainless-steel (Figure 5-1). Stent implantation following angioplasty may be useful to prevent restenosis and occlusion
in coronary and peripheral arteries. The implantation procedure is
similar to percutaneous transluminal angioplasty. The stent is con-
strained on a delivery catheter that is guided under fluoroscopy to

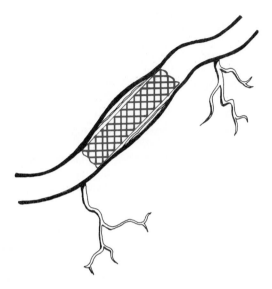

Figure 5-1
Intravascular stent implanted in a coronary artery.

the lesion. Once the location is verified, the constraining membrane is removed to allow the stent to expand. Stent occlusion, bleeding resulting from anticoagulation, or cardiac tamponade related to coronary artery dissection are major complications. Emergent CABG surgery is also a possibility for patients undergoing stent placement.

Transluminal Atherectomy

Transluminal atherectomy is a nonsurgical procedure that removes atheromatous deposits from arteries. The patient is taken to the cardiac catheterization laboratory where an atherectomy catheter is guided percutaneously to the stenotic area. The atheroma is shaved off the vessel wall and collected in the catheter. The catheter balloon is inflated (without dilating the stenosis) to stabilize the cylindrical tube that is used to cut and retrieve the atheroma (Figure 5-2). The procedure is repeated until the obstruction is reduced. Patients should receive heparin during the procedure. Complications

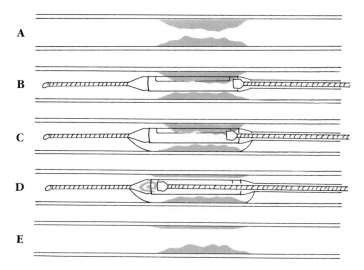

Figure 5-2
Atherectomy procedure. **A**, Identified lesion. **B**, Catheter guided across the lesion. **C**, Balloon inflated to stabilize the catheter. **D**, Cutter is advanced (specimen is trapped in the cylindrical housing). **E**, Balloon is deflated and catheter is removed.
Modified from Simpson J, et al: *Am J Cardiol* 61:97G, 1988.

may include acute occlusion of the vessel, embolus formation, vascular spasm, or vessel perforation. Emergent CABG surgery is a possibility for patients undergoing coronary atherectomy.

Radiofrequency Catheter Ablation

Radiofrequency catheter ablation is a nonsurgical treatment for refractory tachydysrhythmias. Although the technique is used primarily for supraventricular tachycardia (SVT) associated with Wolff-Parkinson-White syndrome (WPW) or atrioventricular (AV) nodal reentry, it also has been used successfully to treat ventricular tachycardia.

Radiofrequency current, delivered to the endocardium via a catheter, is used to destroy or ablate an accessory pathway or dysrythmogenic area that is necessary to sustain the tachycardia. The efficacy of this procedure for SVTs is high and the complication rate is low. Post-procedure care and recovery are similar to that following cardiac catheterization.

Cardiomyoplasty

Patients with low cardiac output who are not candidates for cardiac transplantation may benefit from cardiomyoplasty. This surgical procedure involves wrapping the latissimus dorsi muscle around the heart. The heart is then electrostimulated in synchrony with ventricular systole. This procedure improves cardiac output and organ perfusion and may reduce medication requirements and future hospitalizations. Inotropic and vasopressor agents are administered postoperatively to maintain cardiac output until the pulse generator is activated (within 2 to 3 weeks). Immediate postoperative care is similar to that of any cardiac surgery patient. Since the muscle flap obliterates the left upper lobe and can reduce vital capacity by as much as 20%, aggressive pulmonary hygiene is imperative. An exercise regimen to benefit the left upper extremity may be prescribed during the second postoperative week.

Circulatory Assist Devices

Circulatory assist devices improve tissue perfusion and maintain systemic circulation in patients in cardiogenic shock unresponsive to pharmacologic agents and counterpulsation, patients who cannot be weaned from cardiopulmonary bypass, and those with severe ventricular dysfunction who are awaiting cardiac transplantation.

Several circulatory assist devices are available. Right-sided and/or left-sided ventricular assist devices (VADs) may be used to reroute blood from the native ventricle, so that preload and afterload are reduced in the failing heart. Blood flows through the device and is returned via a cannula placed into the aorta or femoral artery. Patients should receive heparin while dependent upon the VAD, which places the patient at risk for bleeding. In addition, blood cell damage and right ventricular failure (associated with a left VAD) can occur. Cardiac tamponade, air emboli or thrombus formation, sepsis, renal failure, and respiratory failure can also develop. Mechanical failure of the device is also a possibility.

Emergency situations include exsanguination resulting from tubing disconnection or cannulae dislodgment and cardiac arrest. External cardiac compressions are contraindicated; however, internal cardiac massage and defibrillation can be performed.

The patient is taken to the operating room for insertion of the VAD. Hemodynamic improvement should begin within 48 hours. To wean patients from a VAD, the device is turned off for trial periods while carefully assessing hemodynamic progress.

The HeartMate is a heart assist device that is implanted in the abdomen and connected to an external air power supply. This circulatory assist device is portable and allows the patient to be disconnected from the console for short periods of time. Thus the HeartMate allows patients to improve their physical condition while awaiting heart transplantation.

A less invasive assist device used to treat patients with cardiogenic shock secondary to acute MI is the HEMOPUMP. The HEMOPUMP is generally inserted in the femoral artery where the cannula is advanced to the left ventricle. The pump is positioned in the descending aorta and is powered by a motor outside the body attached to a drive cable. The pump's turbine blade spins at a high velocity and draws oxygenated blood out of the left ventricle, reducing afterload and allowing the ventricle time to rest and recover.

Total Artificial Heart

The artificial heart is a last resort in treatment for the failing heart and is currently approved as a bridge to heart transplantation.

The prosthetic ventricles contain diaphragms lubricated with graphite and are controlled by a pneumatically driven system. The drive system can control heart rate, right and left drive pressures, percent systole, and vacuum. Cardiac outputs and ventricular filling pressures of the right and left ventricles can be monitored, in addition to the systolic drive pressures (pressures necessary to eject blood during systole).

Electrical activity does not exist in an artificial heart, therefore dysrhythmias are not a problem. However, the artificial heart does not exist without complications. Thrombus formation may develop with embolization to the brain, kidney, liver, and other organs. Anticoagulation therapy with heparin is required, thus hemorrhage is a major concern. Infection is another problem, since the drive lines provide a direct access to the thoracic cavity. Blood cells may be damaged by the artificial heart and result in anemia, impaired clotting, and infection. Renal failure, seizures, and pulmonary insufficiency are also potential complications. Mechanical failure is always a possibility, so a backup system should be available. Research is being conducted on battery-operated artificial hearts that are totally implantable, eliminating the need for pneumatic tubes, external consoles, and power sources.

Selected bibliography

Abou-Awdi N: Thermo cardiosystems left ventricular assist device as a bridge to cardiac transplant, *AACN Clinical Issues in Critical Care Nursing* 2(3):545-21, 1991.

Bevans M, McLimore E: Intracoronary stents: a new approach to coronary artery dilatation, *Journal of Cardiovasc Nursing* 7(1): 34-49, 1992.

Chiu RJ, editor: *Biomechanical cardiac assist: cardiomyoplasty and muscle powered devices,* Mt Kisco, NY, 1986, Futura.

Eton D, Ahn S: Trends in endovascular surgery, *Critical Care Nursing Clinics of North America* 3(3):535-549, 1991.

Fulterman L: Cardiac transplantation: a comprehensive nursing perspective (part I), *Heart and Lung* 17(5):499-509, 1988.

Fulterman L: Cardiac transplantation: a comprehensive nursing perspective (part II), *Heart and Lung* 17(6):631-638, 1988.

Grines C, DeMaria A: Optimal utilization of thrombolytic therapy for acute myocardial Infarction: concepts and controversies, *Journal of the American College of Cardiology* 16(1): 223-231, 1990.

Hurst JW, editor: *The heart, arteries, and veins,* New York, 1990, McGraw-Hill.

Kinney M, Packa D, Dunbar S: *AACN's clinical reference for critical care nursing,* ed 3, New York, 1993, McGraw-Hill.

Kirkland L, Taylor R: Pericardiocentesis, *Critical Care Clinics* 8(4):699-712, 1992.

Kuck K, Schluter M: Radiofrequency catheter ablation of accessory pathways, *PACE* 15:1380-1386, September, 1992.

Marchetta S, Stennis E: Ventricular assist devices: application for critical care. *Journal of Cardiovascular Nursing* 2(2):39-51, 1988.

Muirhead J: Heart and heart-lung transplantation, *Critical Care Nursing Clinics of North America* 4(1): 97-109 1992.

Quaal S: Cardiac assist devices, *AACN Clinical Issues in Critical Care Nursing* 2(3):475-605, 1991.

Randall E: Recognizing cardiac tamponade, *Journal of Cardiovascular Nursing* 3(3):42-51, 1989.

Sakallaris B: Laser therapy for cardiovascular disease, *Heart and Lung* 16(5):465-471, 1987.

Sanborn T: Laser angioplasty: what has been learned from experimental studies and clinical trials, *Circulation* 78(3):769-774, 1988.

Special report. Report of the joint ISFC/WHO task force on coronary angioplasty, *Circulation* 78(3):780-789, 1988.

Speroni R, and others: Coronary atherectomy: overview and implications for nursing, *Journal of Cardiovascular Nursing* 7(1):25-33, 1992.

Swearingen P, Keen J, editors: *Manual of critical care,* St Louis, 1991, Mosby.

Health Promotion and Home Care

6

Patient Education

To facilitate patient and family adaptation to changes in life-style and compliance with the therapeutic regimen, health care professionals assume an important role in educating the patient and family during the acute phase of hospitalization and in extending the teaching-learning process after the patient is discharged from the hospital.

Learning Needs

The need for learning must be identified and validated. Learning can be described as the difference between what should be (knowledge and skills necessary to maintain or improve cardiovascular function) and what is (the patient's actual knowledge and skill level). Needs vary from individual to individual and can change throughout the patient's acute hospitalization and rehabilitative phases.

Learner Assessment

Validation of the learning need is an important first step in the teaching-learning process. Assessment of the patient as "learner" is equally important. This assessment should include the patient's perception of the illness or condition; response to the illness or condition; beliefs and values of health and illness; history of previous compliance; daily routines, habits, and employment; support system; economic status; home situation, environment, and com-

251

munity resources; educational level; and physical and sensory limitations.

Barriers to learning include lack of sleep, pain, fever, fatigue, distractions, some medications (e.g., tranquilizers), fear, lack of financial support, disabilities, value conflicts, and lack of mutual respect and trust between the patient and the health care professional. Since a comprehensive assessment is not feasible in one interactional encounter, collaboration and communication with other health care professionals is necessary to obtain a complete data base from which the patient's strengths and weaknesses can be identified.

Compliance

The patient's acquisition of knowledge does not guarantee compliance with the therapeutic regimen. Failure to follow the prescribed medical regimen may be related to a number of factors.

Limitations of the Health Belief Model* have been recognized, yet it is still used to predict patient compliance. Patients are more likely to comply if they believe they are susceptible to an illness that could have serious effects on their health and family, that certain actions reduce the possibility of contracting the illness, and that those actions are less threatening than the illness. Therefore asking the patient the following questions may provide insight into the likelihood of compliance with the therapeutic regimen: What does this illness mean to you? What effect will it have on you and your family? How do you think this therapy will help you? Do you foresee any problems with this regimen?

Other cues to noncompliance can be obtained from patient assessment and include past history of noncompliance, variability in daily routines, lack of social and financial support, level of stress in the home, and a history of depression. Table 6-1 lists potential problems the health care professional may encounter in patients who do not adhere to their therapeutic regimen. The listed actions are not all inclusive.

Teaching-Learning Plan

Patients who ask questions about their disease or show interest in the nurse's activities are demonstrating a readiness to learn. Gener-

*From Becker MH and others: A new approach to explaining sick-role behavior in low-income populations, *American Journal of Public Health* 64:205-216, 1974.

⋊ Table 6-1   **Patient problems influencing compliance**

Patient Problem	Suggested Actions
Forgetfulness with medications	Provide written instructions. Develop a medication calendar or use an egg carton to dispense pills. Correlate medication taking with certain routines (e.g., brushing teeth, TV shows). Contact patient by phone periodically to reinforce the importance of taking medication, explain the dangers of stopping the medication, and provide positive feedback. Encourage participation of the family and other support systems in patient care.
Confusion	Simplify the regimen when possible. Color-code medication bottles, caps, and directions. Include family and other support systems in care of patient. Contact patient by phone periodically to assess the situation; confusion may be a side effect of drug therapy or electrolyte imbalance.
Medication side effects	Contact physician—dosages may need to be lowered, or medication may need to be changed. Review medication history and use of over-the-counter drugs for possible causes of adverse reactions.
Regimen perceived as complex	Help patient list "do's" and "don'ts" of the regimen; tailor the regimen to the patient's daily activities. Prioritize regimen, and slowly add behaviors. Encourage family and other support systems in care of patient. Contact patient by phone periodically to assess situation.

Continued.

Table 6-1   **Patient problems influencing compliance—cont'd**

Patient Problem	Suggested Actions
Difficulty with diet	Provide list of acceptable favorite foods; list common foods to avoid. Provide sample menus and recipes; involve the individual responsible for purchasing groceries and cooking the meals in the teaching-learning process.
Lack of financial support	Contact physician for possible change of medications to generic version. Ask patient to explore transportation options with neighbors, church, and other organizations.
Impaired physical dexterity	Request flip-top caps on medication bottles. Refer patient to physical therapist for possible aids to assist the patient.
Sensory and language deficit	Provide written instructions for the patient to refer to. Include family and other support systems in teaching-learning process. Explore ways to reduce impairment, (e.g., use of magnifying glass or large print, prescribing liquid medication if swallowing is a problem).

ally, the more educated individuals are, the more motivated they tend to be. Involve patients as active participants. Ask for input in the care plan to increase patient responsibility in the learning process. Discuss risk factor(s) the patient wants to modify. This allows the patient some control and autonomy, which is more acceptable to the patient than being told to change. The many life-style changes associated with improving cardiovascular health can be overwhelming. Thus the teaching-learning process should occur over time; the patient should not be expected to learn everything during the hospitalization period.

Assessment of the patient as learner is ongoing and provides the data for developing the teaching-learning plan. The plan includes the following components: overall goal, learner objectives and outcomes, content, instructional strategies, and learner evaluation methods.

The overall goal gives direction to the teacher and learner and is based on mutually identified need. Learner objectives are deduced from this goal and are specific expectations or outcomes of the learner. The objectives represent the cognitive, affective, or psychomotor domains. What information should be taught flows from the learner objectives; instructional strategies include a variety of methods and tools to facilitate learning and are based on learner characteristics and objectives, learning domains, and resources of time and money. Finally, learner outcomes must be evaluated. Evaluation can be done by oral questioning, pre- and post-test, and/or observation of a return demonstration. These evaluation methods must measure learner outcome achievement. See Table 6-2 for a sample teaching-learning plan based on the learner's need and assessment.

Learner Outcomes

Learning behaviors, referred to as outcomes or objectives, have been divided into three domains and are ordered from simple to complex. These domains influence the choice of teaching strategies as well as evaluation methods. The cognitive domain comprises intellectual behavior; the affective domain concerns attitudes and values, the psychomotor domain addresses motor skills. Any or all of the three domains can be part of a teaching plan.

Instructional Strategies, Methods, and Tools

Common teaching strategies and methods include lecture, discussion, demonstration, or questioning. Teaching-learning sessions can combine strategies to teach individuals and small groups regardless of the learner outcome domain.

Tools available to enhance learning include preprinted materials (e.g., pamphlets and programmed instruction kits) and audiovisual aids (e.g., models or videotapes). All tools should be evaluated by the teacher for accuracy and appropriateness.

Set and Closure

Creating set and achieving closure are two techniques that should be implemented by the teacher regardless of domain or teaching strategy. Creating set is defined as providing the learner with an explanation of what is to come, providing a means to reduce any

Table 6-2 Sample teaching-learning plan

Outcomes	Content	Strategies	Evaluation
Goal: Safe Administration of Digoxin			
List the signs and symptoms of digoxin toxicity (cognitive)	Cardiac and noncardiac signs and symptoms of toxicity	Lecture-discussion, questioning, pamphlet	Post-test or verbal question: Which of the following is a sign of digoxin toxicity? a. Blood in urine b. Pneumonia c. Change in heart rate or rhythm
Accurately take pulse (psychomotor; cognitive also involved)	Sites of pulses, finger placement, calculating heart rate	Lecture, demonstration, chart for calculating rate, diagram of pulse sites and finger placement	Return demonstration taking radial pulse with 100% accuracy
Accept digoxin as a life-long therapy (affective; cognitive also involved)	Effects of digoxin, consequences of missing digoxin or taking too much	Lecture-discussion, questioning: What effects might you expect if you forgot to take your digoxin with you on vacation?	Questioning: What would you do if you felt nauseated after taking your digoxin or found that your prescription ran out?

learner anxiety, and helping the learner view and approach the learning situation in a given way. Achieving closure involves summarizing and reviewing what has been taught, combining the new information with previous knowledge, and applying it to future situations. Closure provides the learner with a sense of accomplishment and satisfaction.

Evaluation of the Teaching-Learning Process

Evaluation of learner outcome achievement and the teaching-learning plan should be ongoing, so that successful behaviors may be reinforced in the learner and corrective action taken once the strengths and weaknesses of the plan have been identified. A successful teaching-learning process includes attainment of learner outcomes and competent teaching. Success of teaching and learning depends on a number of factors. Thus a reassessment of the components of the teaching-learning process is essential to identify the cause(s) of the failure. A diagram summarizing the teaching-learning process is located in the box on p. 258.

Documentation of Patient Education

Document the teaching plan as well as the patient's response (learning) to the plan in the patient's medical chart. Record the patient's questions and progress, classes attended, and printed materials received. Document the degree of learner outcome achievement and any referrals made to enhance the learning process. Provide continuity of teaching by providing the patient with a copy of the teaching plan and forwarding a copy to the appropriate agency or cardiac rehabilitation program. Family or other support system involvement in the teaching-learning process should also be documented.

Conclusion

Patient education is a responsibility of health care professionals and requires active patient participation.

Teaching plans give direction to both the learner and the teacher. Brief teaching sessions can be carried out while performing other health-related activities.

Reinforce learning, but avoid duplication of teaching. Communicate the plan to other health care professionals, and document the teaching sessions and the degree of learner outcome achievement.

Overview of the Teaching-Learning Process

Assessment
- Learning need

Validation of Need
- Verification of knowledge deficit

Assessment of Learner
- Perception of illness
- Response to illness
- Health/illness beliefs
- Previous compliance history
- Routines, habits, employment
- Support systems
- Home, environment, community
- Economic status
- Educational level
- Physical/sensory limitations

Prediction of Problems

Prediction of Strengths

Identification of Barriers

Development of Plan
- Overall goal
- Learner outcomes
- Content
- Instructional strategies, methods, tools
- Learner evaluation tool

Implement Plan
- Create set
- Achieve closure

Evaluation of
          Teaching-Learning Process

          ↙   ↘

Unsuccessful   Successful
- Outcomes not met   - Outcomes met
- Teaching ineffective   - Teaching effective

Teaching may be necessary after the patient is discharged from the hospital, requiring other health care professionals to assume responsibility for the continuity of health education of cardiovascular patients and their families.

Core Curriculum for the Cardiovascular Patient

Teaching the patient and family about the heart and vascular system is imperative in the prevention and treatment of cardiovascular disease. The following pages present an outline of core cardiovascular information that can be tailored to address individualized patient or family needs as well as specific physician instructions.

1. Basic anatomy and physiology

    Brief description of structure and function of heart and vessels.

2. Pathophysiology

    Brief description of oxygen supply and demand concept, atherosclerosis, specific patient problem (e.g., coronary artery disease, congestive heart failure, valve disease, peripheral vascular disease).

3. Major cardiac reasons to consult physician

    Angina—temporary pain, usually precipitated by physical activity, emotional stress, heavy meals, sexual activity, extreme cold or heat.

    Instructions—rest, place nitroglycerin under tongue (one every 5 minutes—maximum of three tablets) or use aerosol nitroglycerin (one premeasured dose every 5 minutes—maximum of three doses); if pain is not relieved, call physician or go immediately to an emergency room. Time is a critical factor in the success of treatment; do not delay seeking help.

    Myocardial Infarction—prolonged pain, often occurring at rest and lasting more than 5 minutes, not relieved by rest or nitroglycerin; associated symptoms include sweating, shortness of breath, weakness, nausea, and vomiting.

    Instructions—call Emergency Medical System (EMS) or go immediately to an emergency room. Time is a critical factor in the success of treatment; do not delay seeking help.

    Congestive Heart Failure—unusual fatigue, shortness of breath, inability to sleep lying flat, swelling of the feet or ankles, a weight gain of more than 2 to 3 pounds in 1 day (weigh at same time each day with same amount of clothing and after urination), frequent urination at night, persistent cough.

    Instructions—call physician, practice preventive measures, (e.g., adhere to salt restriction in diet) and take medications as prescribed (diuretics and digitalis).

4. Risk factors and suggested modification

Nonmodifiable—cannot be changed

- Age
- Gender (males are at greater risk than females)
- Heredity

Modifiable—can be controlled or eliminated

- Smoking—stop smoking (community resources are available)
- High blood pressure (hypertension)—control weight, limit dietary salt intake, exercise, take medication if prescribed
- High blood fat level (hyperlipidemia)—alter diet to achieve:

    Cholesterol ≤200 mg/dl (<180 mg/dl if under 30 years of age)

    Triglycerides ≤500 mg/dl (ideally <250 mg/dl)

    Take medication (if prescribed)
- Diabetes—diet to control blood sugar, control weight, exercise, medication (if prescribed)
- Obesity—decrease caloric intake, exercise, modify eating behaviors
- Physical inactivity—exercise regularly (consult physician about type and extent of activity)
- Stress—exercise, practice relaxation techniques (biofeedback, meditation, behavior modification, and yoga)

5. Diet

Some risk factors associated with diet include overweight, elevated serum lipids, and high blood pressure; a diet will be prescribed by the dietitian. Guidelines for promoting cardiovascular health include the following:

- Reduce fat and cholesterol intake; emphasize a diet rich in grains, fruits, vegetables, legumes. Limit intake of cholesterol to <300 mg/day, even less if cholesterol is elevated. Avoid foods high in cholesterol, including eggs, dairy products, organ meats, and fatty meats. Limit intake of total fat and saturated fat to <30% of total calories, even less if cholesterol is elevated. Small amounts of polyunsaturated fats are preferred to saturated fats. Recent evidence has shown that olive oil, a monounsaturated fat, may also be beneficial in lowering blood cholesterol. Polyunsaturated fats (liquid at room temperature) include safflower, sunflower, corn, soybean, and cottonseed oils. Saturated fats (most are solid at room temperature) include shortening, lard, cocoa butter, coconut oil, and palm oil. Monounsaturated fats include olive oil and peanut oil.

· Reduce triglyceride intake (if applicable). Achieve and maintain ideal weight; limit alcohol intake; reduce fat intake to <30% of total caloric intake; substitute complex carbohydrates (starches and fiber) for simple carbohydrates (e.g., candy and desserts).

· Reduce sodium intake. Table salt, or sodium chloride, is 40% sodium. Most people need only the equivalent of 1/10 teaspoon of salt per day. Do not add salt when cooking or eating; avoid obviously salty foods such as chips, bacon, or cold cuts. Avoid canned soups, vegetables, and condiments (e.g., catsup, mustard, soy sauce). Eat homemade broths and fresh vegetables; season food with herbs and spices (powders, not salts).

· Maintain ideal weight. Eat a balanced, low-calorie diet, modify eating behaviors, and exercise regularly.

· Read labels; the item listed first is the major ingredient of the product. To meet nutritional criteria for cardiovascular health, restricted items such as salt should be absent or appear toward the end of the ingredient list.

6. Medications   (See Tables 6-3 to 6-10, pp. 264-276, for teaching guidelines related to specific cardiovascular medications; see Chapter 4 for more information on cardiovascular medications.)

Medication Basics—For each medication discuss name, dosage, frequency, route, purpose, major side effects, major interactions with foods and other drugs, and special factors (e.g., pulse limitations).

Storage Instructions—Store in a cool, dry place away from direct heat; recommended storage temperature is 15° to 30° C (59° to 86° F), unless otherwise specified.

Keep out of reach of children.

Discard outdated medication; discard medication not currently prescribed.

Schedule for Taking Medication—Write out a schedule for taking medication(s), keeping it as simple as possible.

Missed Dose—Take as soon as remembered if not close to the next scheduled dose; do not take a double dose. If you cannot remember if you took a dose, wait until the next scheduled time to take the medication.

Other General Information—Do not crush or chew sustained release products.

Do not take over-the-counter (OTC) medications without physician approval.

Do not take medicine prescribed for someone else.

Do not stop taking your medication without physician approval.

Report side effects to your physician.

Keep plenty of prescribed medications on hand; remember that you may not be able to fill prescriptions on weekends, holidays, or vacations.

7. General activity

Consult physician regarding returning to work, leisure activities, and driving. General guidelines include:

Get up and get dressed each morning.

Perform self-care activities as usual (e.g., bathing and shaving).

Pace activities; plan rest periods.

Walk up and down stairs at a comfortable pace.

Avoid: Straining or lifting—>10 pounds after surgery, >30 pounds after myocardial infarction. Exercises such as pushups or pullups. Excessive straining with bowel movements. Crossing legs and activities that may kink peripheral bypass grafts (PVOD patients).

Walk outside, weather permitting; walking should be the primary physical activity until the first follow-up visit to the physician.

Limit visitors and phone calls initially to prevent fatigue.

Be aware of warnings to stop exercise or activity:
  · Chest pain or pressure (other than from surgical incision)
  · Shortness of breath
  · Dizziness or faintness
  · Unusual weakness or fatigue

8. Sexual activity

Follow physician instructions. General guidelines include:

Be well rested before engaging in sexual activity.

Wait 1 to 2 hours after eating.

Use a comfortable position.

Provide for a comfortable environment, avoiding temperature extremes.

Avoid sexual activity with an unfamiliar partner.

Rest afterward.

Do not use alcohol or recreational drugs prior to sexual activity.

Use nitroglycerin prophylactically (with physician approval).

Be aware of these symptoms and consult physician if they occur:

- Angina during or after intercourse
- Sleeplessness or unusual fatigue the following day
- Increased heart rate and respirations that continue 20 minutes after sexual activity

Possible reasons for sexual dysfunction in the cardiovascular patient include medication, anxiety, depression, fatigue, fear of failure, and decreased vasocongestion caused by peripheral vascular occlusive disease.

9. Psychosocial concerns

Depression, fear, and anxiety—These emotions are common, usually temporary, reactions to myocardial infarction or cardiovascular surgery; encourage patient to discuss emotions; encourage patient to be as active as the physician allows; refer to physician, clergy, psychologist, or social worker.

Finances—Refer to financial counselor or social worker.

Self-care and home management—Refer to social worker, Visiting Nurse Association, and other community resources (e.g., Mended Hearts, Meals on Wheels, smoking cessation programs, and weight management programs). Learning needs commonly change after discharge from the hospital as patients realize they must care for themselves. Knowledge of available resources can be a great comfort.

10. Incisions (surgical patients)

Wash gently with soap and water; do not scrub.

Numbness, soreness, itching, redness, and mild swelling will gradually disappear.

Maintain good posture, move about despite incisional discomfort.

Take prescribed pain medication if needed.

Call physician if the following occurs:

· Excessive swelling
· New or increased drainage
· Foul-smelling drainage
· Unusual tenderness
· New or increased redness
· Onset of fever

11. Follow-up care

Call physician's office for a follow-up appointment or special instructions (e.g., lab work prior to office visit or suture removal).

12. Taking of pulse

Instruct patient on taking pulse (radial or carotid with physician approval) to monitor response to activity or medications and assess pacemaker function.

Table 6-3   **Patient education guidelines for antianginal agents**

Antianginal agents are prescribed to reduce the demand and workload on the heart and to improve blood flow via the coronary arteries to the myocardium.

Directions	
Nitrates	Short-acting nitrates should be taken at the first sign of angina, then every 5 minutes until pain is relieved, up to three doses. If the pain is not relieved, the patient should go to the nearest emergency room or medical facility.
Sublingual	Do not swallow sublingual nitroglycerin; let it dissolve under the tongue. Remove cotton from the nitroglycerin container; keep tablets in the original glass container. Replace sublingual tablets every 6 months.
Aerosol	Nitroglycerin can be sprayed on or under the tongue; do not shake the container and do not inhale the spray.

Table 6-3   **Patient education guidelines for antianginal agents—cont'd**

Oral	Long-acting nitrates should be taken with one glass of water 1 hour before or 2 hours after meals for faster absorption.
Buccal	Buccal dosage forms should be placed between the upper lip and gum and allowed to dissolve. Avoid buccal dosage form at bedtime (aspiration may result).
Ointment	Spread over a 2×3 inch area. Do not rub or massage area. Apply to a hairless area. Remove old ointment before applying new dose. Rotate site frequently.
Transdermal	Do not cut or trim the patch; apply on a hairless area. Avoid placing patch below the knee or elbow. If patch becomes loose or falls off, replace with a new transdermal dosage form. Rotate sites frequently.
Beta adrenergic blocking agents	Beta adrenergic blocking agents can be taken with food or on an empty stomach. Check pulse; if <50 bpm, call physician before taking medication.
Calcium channel blocking agents	Calcium channel blocking agents (except nifedipine and nicardipine) can slow the heart rate. Check pulse; if <50 bpm call physician before taking medication. Nifedipine capsules may be punctured and administered sublingually or buccally.
Missed Dose	Do not take a double dose of antianginal agents.
Nitrates	Take dose as soon as remembered if it is more than 2 hours before the next scheduled dose, or more than 6 hours before the next scheduled dose of an extended release dosage form.

Continued.

Table 6-3   **Patient education guidelines for antianginal agents—cont'd**

Beta adrenergic blocking agents	Take dose as soon as remembered if it is more than 4 hours before the next scheduled dose (8 hours if taking atenolol, labetalol, nadolol, and extended release propranolol).
Calcium channel blocking agents	Take dose as soon as possible unless it is almost time for the next scheduled dose.
Cautions	Do not stop taking medication without physician approval. Hot weather and hot tub baths may enhance hypotensive effects. Stop smoking. Dizziness may pose a safety problem. Although you may feel well, do not overexert.
Nitrates	Rise slowly after taking nitroglycerin.
Calcium channel blocking agents	Use good dental and oral hygiene if taking calcium channel blocking agents.
Drug-Drug Interactions	Avoid OTC medications unless approved by a physician. Alcohol can enhance hypotensive effects. Antianginal agents may react with other prescribed medications. Discuss all your medications with a health care professional.
Side Effects	Report the following to physician: fainting, severe dizziness, chest pain or discomfort, breathing difficulty, slow or fast heart rate, weight gain, swelling in ankles or feet, prolonged headache.
Beta adrenergic blocking agents	Cold extremities, fever, sore throat, mental depression, or peripheral cyanosis.
Calcium channel blocking agents	Overgrowth of gums.

Table 6-4   **Patient education guidelines for antidysrhythmic agents**

Antidysrhythmic medications are prescribed to control abnormal heart rate or rhythm. Beta adrenergic blocking agents and calcium channel blocking agents are discussed in Table 6-3.

Directions	Take the exact amount prescribed at evenly spaced intervals.
	Verapamil, beta blockers: Check pulse to determine rhythm and heart rate; contact physician if <50 bpm.
	Procainamide, quinidine, mexiletine, tocainide, and beta blockers: May be taken with food.
	Disopyramide: Take 1 hour before or 2 hours after eating. Ice, sugarless candy, or gum will help relieve dry mouth.
Missed Dose	Do not take a double dose of antidysrhythmics.
	Procainamide, quinidine: Take the missed dose only if remembered within 2 hours.
	Encainide, mexiletine, disopyramide, propafenone, moricizine, tocainide: Take the missed dose only if remembered within 4 hours.
	Flecainide: Take the missed dose only if remembered within 6 hours.
	Amiodarone: If two or more doses are missed, contact physician.
Cautions	Visual disturbances or dizziness may pose a safety problem. Do not stop taking this medication without physician approval.
	Amiodarone: Protect skin from sunlight; use barrier sun block and protective clothing. Side effects may continue months after drug is discontinued.

Continued.

Table 6-4   **Patient education guidelines for antidysrhythmic agents—cont'd**

Drug-Drug Interactions	Antidysrhythmic agents may react with other prescribed medications. Discuss all medications with a health care professional. Avoid OTC medications unless approved by a physician.
Side Effects	Report the following to physician: change in heart rate or rhythm, chest pain, blurred vision, severe dizziness or lightheadedness, shortness of breath, fever, chills, diarrhea, numbness, tingling, weight gain or swelling of ankles or feet.
	Tocainide, flecainide, mexiletine, procainamide, or quinidine: bruising or bleeding.
	Amiodarone: blue-gray skin discoloration, cough, painful or difficult breathing, difficulty in walking, weakness, yellow skin or eyes.

Table 6-5   **Patient education guidelines for digoxin**

Digoxin is prescribed to improve pumping action of the heart or control abnormal heart rate and rhythm.

Directions	Take the exact amount prescribed. Check pulse; if pulse <60 bpm, or a change in rhythm is noticed, contact physician before taking digoxin. Take with or between meals.
Missed Dose	Do not take a double dose. If more than 12 hours before the next scheduled dose, take the missed dose. Contact physician if digoxin has not been taken in 2 or more days.

Table 6-5   **Patient education guidelines for digoxin—cont'd**

Cautions	Adhere to prescribed diet while taking this medication. Do not stop taking the medication without physician approval. Any change in medication regimen can potentially affect digitalis serum level.
Drug-Drug Interactions	Avoid OTC medications unless approved by a physician. Avoid taking digoxin with antacids, laxatives, cholestyramine, or colestipol. Digoxin may react with other prescribed medications. Discuss all medications with a health care professional.
Side Effects	Report the following to physician: loss of appetite, nausea and vomiting, extreme weakness or fatigue, change in heart rate or rhythm, visual disturbances, weight gain, swelling of ankles or feet.

Table 6-6   **Patient education guidelines for diuretic agents**

Diuretics are prescribed to rid the body of excess fluid.

Directions	Take the exact amount prescribed. May be taken with food. Take early in the day to avoid waking during the night to urinate.
Missed Dose	Do not take a double dose of diuretics. Take the missed dose as soon as remembered, and if it is not too close to the next scheduled dose.
Cautions	Adhere to prescribed diet; limit sodium intake. Do not stop taking this medi-

Continued.

Table 6-6   Patient education guidelines for diuretic agents—cont'd

	cation without physician approval. Rise slowly from a sitting or supine position. Weakness, muscle cramps, thirst, or dry mucous membranes may be a sign of electrolyte imbalance and dehydration. Hot weather and diarrhea can predispose you to dehydration. Take potassium supplements as prescribed along with your diuretic. With potassium-sparing diuretic agents, avoid foods high in potassium (e.g., bananas, oranges, avocados, broccoli) and avoid salt substitutes.
Drug-Drug Interactions	Avoid OTC medications unless approved by a physician. Alcohol enhances the hypotensive effects. Patients taking digoxin are at risk for toxic effects when taking a diuretic. Taking diuretics and other medications to control high blood pressure can enhance hypotensive effects. Discuss all medications with a health care professional.
Side Effects	Report the following to physician: increased thirst, dry mucous membranes, dry mouth, weakness, weak pulse, muscle cramps, nausea or vomiting, stomach pain, change in heart rhythm, weight gain, swelling of the ankles or feet, bleeding, bruising.

Table 6-7 **Patient education guidelines for antihypertensive agents**

Antihypertensive agents are prescribed to control high blood pressure. Beta adrenergic blocking agents and calcium channel blocking agents are discussed in Table 6-3

Directions	Take the exact amount prescribed. Record blood pressures; if systolic BP <90 mm Hg, contact physician. Most can be taken with meals. ACE inhibitors should be taken on an empty stomach. *Minoxidil:* Check pulse and daily weight before taking minoxidil; if resting pulse is >20 beats above normal or weight gain is >5 pounds, notify physician. *Clonidine, prazosin, guanfacine, and guanabenz:* Take at bedtime. Sugarless candy or gum or ice may help relieve dry mouth associated with many antihypertensive agents. Transdermal patches should not be trimmed; apply to clean hairless skin on upper arm or upper body. Keep in place while in shower or swimming. Replace patch if it becomes loose or falls off.
Missed Dose	Do not take a double dose of an antihypertensive agent. Take dose as soon as remembered unless it is almost time for the next scheduled dose. Contact physician if two or more oral doses are missed or if 3 days lapse without changing the transdermal patch.

Continued.

Table 6-7   Patient education guidelines for antihypertensive agents—cont'd

Cautions	Adhere to prescribed diet; avoid sodium intake. Do not stop taking the medication without physician approval because blood pressure may rise to dangerously high levels.
	Avoid OTC medications unless approved by a physician.
	Rise slowly from a sitting or supine position.
	Hot weather and hot tub baths can enhance hypotensive effects.
	Dizziness or drowsiness can pose a safety problem.
Drug-Drug Interactions	Antihypertensive agents can react with other prescribed medications. Discuss all your medications with a health care professional.
	Alcohol can enhance hypotensive effects.
	Some OTC medications can interfere with the antihypertensive effects.
Side Effects	Report the following to physician: severe dizziness, fainting, weakness, chest pain, shortness of breath, difficulty breathing, weight gain, swelling of ankles or feet, irregular heart rhythm, fast or slowed heart rate, numbness, tingling of extremities, mental depression, fever, chills, or sore throat.
	Hydralazine: Blisters, general weakness, joint pain, or sore throat.
	Minoxidil: Excessive hair growth.
	Clonidine: Skin irritation or itching with transdermal system; cold, pale fingertips or toes.

Table 6-8   **Patient education guidelines for antihyperlipidemic agents**

Antihyperlipidemic agents are prescribed to lower cholesterol levels and retard the atherosclerotic process.

Directions	*Clofibrate, niacin, probucol:* Take with meals.
	Cholestyramine and colestipol: Take at least 8 hours after digoxin. Take any other medications 6 to 8 hours before cholestyramine or colestipol.
	Colestipol or cholestyramine: Allow powder to sit on liquid (soup or juice) for 1 or 2 minutes; then mix thoroughly (it will not dissolve); drink the solution; rinse the glass with liquid and drink the remaining medication.
	Lovastatin: Take with meals.
Missed Dose	Do not take a double dose.
	Do not take the missed dose if it is close to the next scheduled dose.
Cautions	Adhere to prescribed low-cholesterol diet.
	Diet should include high levels of bulk and fiber to avoid constipation.
	Do not stop taking the medication without physician approval.
Drug-Drug Interactions	Antihyperlipidemic agents interfere with many medications; allow several hours between taking antihyperlipidemic agents and other drugs.
Side Effects	Report the following to physician:
	Clofibrate: Blood in urine, difficult or painful urination, swelling of ankles or feet, chest pain, shortness of breath, diarrhea, nausea or vomiting, stomach pain.

Continued.

Table 6-8   **Patient education guidelines for antihyperlipidemic agents—cont'd**

	Gemfibrozil: Similar to clofibrate.
	Colestipol: Constipation, blood in stool, stomach pain, nausea or vomiting.
	Cholestyramine: Similar to colestipol.
	Niacin: Flushing and itching.
	Lovastatin and Simvastatin: Blurred vision.
	Probucol: Diarrhea, nausea, and abdominal distention with gas.
	All HMG-CoA reductase inhibitors: myalgia

Table 6-9   **Patient education guidelines for hematologic agents**

Hematologic agents are prescribed to decrease clot formation and platelet adhesion.

Directions	These agents may be taken with meals.
	Aspirin: Drink a full glass of fluid and avoid lying down for at least ½ hour after taking aspirin.
	Avoid taking antacids for 1 to 2 hours after taking aspirin.
Missed Dose	Do not take a double dose.
	Take the missed dose as soon as possible if it is not too close to the next scheduled dose.
	Dipyridamole: Can be taken if more than 4 hours before the next scheduled dose.
	Warfarin: Take it as soon as remembered, unless it is the next day.
Cautions	Avoid OTC medications unless approved by a physician.
	Avoid activities that can result in injury.

Table 6-9   **Patient education guidelines for hematologic agents—cont'd**

	Do not stop taking the medication without physician approval.
	Alcohol may enhance bleeding tendencies.
	Wear a Medic Alert bracelet identifying the medication you are taking.
	Let all health care professionals know you are taking an anticoagulant.
	Dipyridamole: Rise slowly from a sitting or supine position.
	Warfarin: Use a soft toothbrush and an electric razor.
Drug-Drug Interactions	Many drugs can interfere with these hematologic agents. Do not take any medication without consulting the physician. Increased risk of bleeding can occur.
Side Effects	Report the following to physician: bleeding gums, unexplained bruising or bleeding, spontaneous nosebleeds, heavy bleeding from cuts or during menstruation, abdominal pain, back pain, joint pain, blood in urine, black stools, blood in sputum, blood in vomit, continued severe headaches, or chest pain.

Table 6-10   **Patient education guidelines for peripheral vascular agents**

Peripheral vascular agents are prescribed to decrease or control symptoms associated with decreased peripheral blood flow.

Directions	These agents can be taken with food.
Missed Dose	Do not take a double dose. Take the dose as soon as it is remembered if it is not close to the next scheduled dose.

Continued.

Table 6-10　**Patient education guidelines for peripheral vascular agents—cont'd**

Cautions	Stop smoking—smoking causes vaso-constriction and aggravates peripheral vascular disease. *Isoxsuprine:* Rise slowly from a sitting or supine position.
Drug-Drug Interactions	Avoid OTC medications unless approved by a physician.
Side Effects	Report the following to physician: chest pain, irregular heart rhythm, faintness, and shortness of breath. *Pentoxifyllin:* Flushing, seizures, and excitement. *Nylidrin:* Blurred vision, difficulty in voiding, metallic taste, fever, and chilliness.

Educating the Patient with Select Cardiovascular Problems and Therapies

The teaching needs for patients with pacemakers, implantable cardioverter defibrillators (ICDs) or patients with peripheral vascular occlusive disease can be found in Tables 6-11 to 6-13.

Cardiac Rehabilitation

Cardiac rehabilitation encompasses patient and family education, physical activity, and psychologic support and counseling. Candidates for rehabilitation range from the patient recovering from cardiac surgery or myocardial infarction to the individual who is interested in reducing risk factors and preventing cardiac problems. Benefits of cardiac conditioning and rehabilitation include improved functional capacity, improved musculoskeletal fitness, and an increased sense of well-being.

An explanation of select cardiac rehabilitation terms begins on p. 282.

Text continued on page 280.

Table 6-11   **Patient education guidelines for pacemakers**

Topics to Review	
Cardiac anatomy and physiology	Brief overview
Information about pacemaker	Sample of lead and generator for patient to look at, if possible; reason for pacemaker; importance of keeping manufacturer's instruction booklet; importance of carrying pacemaker identification card at all times (card may be available prior to discharge or may be mailed to patient); inform patient about Medic-Alert bracelet.
Activity	Generally, no restrictions specific to pacemaker (consult with physician); sexual activity permitted.
Pulse	Check pulse daily; obtain safe pulse range from physician; if pulse is outside of specified range, notify physician.
Site care	Keep incision clean and dry until healed; observe for signs of infection (redness, swelling, drainage, and fever).
Electromagnetic interference	Usually not a problem; if dizziness and other symptoms occur when near a microwave, television or radio transmitter, or airport screening device, move away from source.
Consult physician for:	· Follow-up appointment in office or via transtelephonic monitoring system (learn how to use).
	· Symptoms of dizziness, difficulty breathing, palpitations, chest pain, syncope, and prolonged hiccups.
	· Heart rate outside of specified range.
Personal physician and dentist	Notify of pacemaker implant prior to treatment.

Table 6-12 **Patient education guidelines for implantable cardioverter defibrillators (ICD)**

Topics to Review	
Cardiac anatomy and physiology	Brief overview
Reason for ICD	Include instructions about identification card and wearing Medic-Alert necklace or bracelet.
CPR	Instruct family members to learn CPR. Instruct patient about "cough" CPR (with physician approval)
	If symptoms (faintness or palpitations) occur, cough vigorously once every 2 seconds; continue for 30 seconds.
	If ICD does not discharge in 30 seconds, stop coughing.
	If symptoms continue, call Emergency Medical System (EMS).
Consult physician if	· Swelling or purulent drainage is noted at incision site
	· Fever develops and persists more than 1 day
	· Audible beeping tones are heard from generator
	· If there are ICD discharges (single shock may not require office visit)
Call Emergency Medical System (EMS) if	· ICD discharges more than two times
	· Patient is unstable or symptoms persist after one shock.
Diary	List date, time, warning signs, symptoms, and activity at time of ICD discharge.
Activity	Avoid pressure, manipulation of skin covering generator. Physical activity is acceptable as tolerated, including sexual activity.

Table 6-12   Patient education guidelines for implantable
cardioverter defibrillators (ICD)—cont'd

Precautions	Avoid strong magnetic fields that may activate or deactivate the ICD; do not touch the antenna of a citizen's band radio, spark plug, distributor wire of a running car or lawnmower; avoid the immediate area around a radio or television transmitting tower; avoid use of diathermy or electrocautery treatments. Household appliances such as microwaves, televisions, saws, and other small tools pose no problem to the ICD; airport security scanners will detect ICD but pose no problem.
Driving	Do not drive until physician approves.
Medications	Continue medications as instructed; ICD does not replace the need for antidysrhythmics.
ICD discharge effect on others	Anyone touching a patient implanted with an ICD will feel a small, harmless shock at the time of discharge.
Personal physician and dentist	Notify of ICD implant prior to treatment.

Table 6-13   Patient education guidelines for peripheral
vascular occlusive disease (PVOD)—foot care

Hygiene	Wash feet with warm water daily; dry gently, but thoroughly, especially between the toes; wear clean socks each day (wool or cotton absorb moisture better than nylon).
Temperature	Keep feet warm, avoid extreme heat or cold; exercise caution when using heating pads or bathing to prevent burns (do not exceed 110° F).

Continued.

Table 6-13   **Patient education guidelines for peripheral vascular occlusive disease (PVOD)—foot care—cont'd**

Safety and comfort	Wear comfortable hose and shoes that do not cause undue pressure, especially on toes and heels; avoid causing trauma to the feet—do not walk barefoot or wear open-toed shoes; apply powder if feet perspire; apply lotion if feet are dry; place lamb's wool between toes to keep them dry and prevent rubbing; exercise caution when cutting toenails (a podiatrist can safely provide this service).
Circulation	Do not wear garters or constricting clothing; do not cross legs at knees; place a pillow at foot of bed under covers to prevent top covers from resting on feet.
Consult physician for:	· Breaks in skin, redness, swelling, blisters, pain, or other foot or leg discomfort · Changes in skin color, temperature, and sensation · Permission to use new medications, strong topical agents, and OTC corn remedies.

Cardiac Rehabilitation Phases

The American College of Sports Medicine classifies cardiac rehabilitation into three phases:

Phase I—in hospital, early convalescence

Phase II—immediate postdischarge, transition to return to normal activities

Phase III—recovery, long-term maintenance

The primary objective of phase I is to prevent the patient from becoming deconditioned as a result of physical inactivity. Patients without complications can initiate self-care within the first 1 to 3 days after open heart surgery or myocardial infarction. Progression to range-of-motion exercises, select arm and leg exercises, and

Activity Guidelines

Prior to Activity

* Note cardiac history, e.g., MI, CHF.
* Note hemoglobin and hematocrit values.
* Question the patient concerning most recent activity and response to that activity.
* Be certain the patient is rested.
* Administer pain medication if necessary before activity.
* Obtain BP and HR in a supine or sitting position. Repeat BP reading while patient is standing.
* If patient is on telemetry, notify monitor attendant of activity.
* If supplemental oxygen is ordered while patient is resting, use portable oxygen during activity.

During Activity

* Note response to activity. Abnormal exercise responses are listed in Table 6-14, p. 283.
* Ask patient to quantify difficulty of activity using the Borg Scale (Table 6-16). A rate of perceived exertion (RPE) of 11 or 12 corresponds to a heart rate of approximately 110 to 120 and is appropriate for the hospitalized patient.
* Determine whether activity should be altered (i.e., discontinued or decreased in intensity).

Activity Follow-up

* Obtain BP and HR.
* Document type and extent of activity (e.g., number of feet walked), patient response to activity, BP and HR before and after activity, any significant change in HR/rhythm during activity.

walking can follow quickly based on the patient's tolerance of activity. See Activity Guidelines in the box above. The overall goal is to safely increase the amount of activity so the patient is able to comfortably perform activities requiring 3 to 4 METs by the time of discharge.

In addition to reinforcing patient education and providing continued psychologic support, a major objective of phase II is reversal of deconditioning and initiation of a structured conditioning program. The purpose of phase III is to assist the patient in retaining achievements made in phase II. There is no end point in phase III, since it is a maintenance program. Some patients will continue phase III for months or years, others will elect to implement their own exercise program rather than continuing in a structured phase III program. Research is ongoing to evaluate the effects of regular aerobic activity.

Select Cardiac Rehabilitation Terminology

MET

MET is the unit of measurement for oxygen uptake that approximates 3.5 ml O_2/kg/min, or the oxygen uptake at rest. MET provides a means of predicting the energy expenditure for certain activities. During the acute phase of hospitalization (CCU), energy expenditure is approximately 1.5 to 2 METs. By the time of discharge, patients should be able to perform activities of daily living (ADLs), which require 3 to 4 METs. Table 6-15 discusses METs associated with various activities.

Rate of Perceived Exertion

The rate of perceived exertion (RPE) is the patient's perception of the difficulty of an exercise or activity. The patient rates the difficulty of the activity by selecting the appropriate number on the Borg RPE Scale of 6 to 20 (Table 6-16). The upper limits of the target heart rate (THR) generally correspond to an RPE of 12 to 15. The RPE should not exceed these levels. The value range of 6 to 20 corresponds with heart rates ranging from 60 to 200 bpm. For example, 10 would correspond to a heart rate of approximately 100 bpm. An RPE of 11 or 12 is appropriate for the hospitalized patient. This scale is most commonly used in cardiac rehabilitation programs. It may also be used effectively by patients who are unable to determine an accurate pulse rate or by patients who may have a slower than normal increase in heart rate with activity (e.g., following cardiac transplant).

Exercise Prescription

An exercise prescription is an individualized outline or "prescription" for activity that is ideally based on a graded exercise test. The

Table 6-14   **Abnormal exercise responses***

SBP ↑ >20 mm Hg	SBP ↓ >10 mm Hg
DBP ↓ >10 mm Hg	
HR ↑ >20 bpm	HR ↓ >10 bpm

ST segment change >1 mm elevation or depression during exercise.

Severe dyspnea, angina, or faintness.

PVCs with activity, new atrial fibrillation or "old" atrial fibrillation with HR >120.

*Hospitalized patient following surgery or myocardial infarction.
SBP, Systolic blood pressure; DBP, diastolic blood pressure; HR, heart rate; PVCs, premature ventricular complexes.

Table 6-15   **MET expenditure table***

1-2 MET activities	Lying quietly
	Sitting in a chair
	Eating
	Washing hands or face
	Reading
2-3 MET activities	Dressing or undressing
	Using bedside commode
	Walking around the house
	Fixing a light meal
	Riding in a car
3-4 MET activities	Showering (standing)
	Fixing dinner
	Making bed
	Washing dishes
	Bicycling 5 mph
4-5 MET activities	Using bedpan
	Carrying light objects
	Grocery shopping
	Dancing
	Sexual activity

*Approximate MET levels for a person weighing 70 kg.

Table 6-16   **Borg's RPE Scale (15 grades)**

6	14
7 very, very light	15 hard
8	16
9 very light	17 very hard
10	18
11 fairly light	19 very, very hard
12	20
13 somewhat hard	

From Borg G: *Medicine and Science in Sports and Exercise,* 14:378, 1982.

components of a prescription include frequency of exercise—number of times per week (usually three to five); intensity of exercise—grade (if on treadmill) and speed; duration of exercise—length of time, including warm-up period, aerobic activity, and cool-down period. Warm-up and cool-down periods are important, since they allow the body to gradually get ready for and recover from the more vigorous activity of the aerobic phase of exercise.

Maximum Heart Rate

Maximum heart rate is defined as the heart rate at which highest or maximal oxygen uptake is achieved. It is determined by a graded exercise test or predetermined based on age and physical condition. Maximum heart rate can be estimated by subtracting patient's age from 220 (e.g., a 40-year-old has an estimated maximum heart rate of 180).

Target Heart Rate

Target heart rate (THR) is the heart rate at which desired conditioning effects will be achieved, usually 70% to 85% of maximal heart rate. The goal of aerobic activity is to reach but not exceed the THR. Based on symptoms and cardiac function, some patients may have a THR considerably lower than 70% of maximum.

Isometric Exercise

Isometric exercise is static activity that involves development of tension during muscular contraction with little, if any, change in muscle length or joint movement. Lifting weights, pushups, and carrying heavy objects are examples of isometric exercise. Patients with limited cardiac reserve should avoid isometric exercise.

Isotonic Exercise

Isotonic exercise involves rhythmic, repetitive muscle relaxation and contraction, and joint movement. Walking, jogging, swimming, and bicycling are examples of isotonic exercise. These activities increase aerobic metabolism and contribute to cardiovascular conditioning.

Rate Pressure Product

Rate pressure product (RPP), also known as double product, is the heart rate multiplied by systolic blood pressure (normal is <12,000). The RPP is an index to estimate myocardial oxygen consumption or demand. Activities performed at a lower systolic blood pressure and heart rate (lower RPP) are less likely to create a supply/demand imbalance that causes signs and symptoms in the patient with coronary disease.

Selected bibliography

American Association of Cardiovascular and Pulmonary Rehabilitation: *Guidelines for cardiac rehabilitation programs,* Champaign, IL, 1990, Human Kinetics Books.

Brannon P, Johnson R: The internal cardioverter defibrillator: patient-family teaching, *Focus on Critical Care* 19(1):41-46, 1992.

Braunwald E editor: *Heart disease: a textbook of cardiovascular medicine,* Philadelphia, 1992, WB Saunders.

Karam C: *A practical guide to cardiac rehabilitation,* Rockville, MD, 1989, Aspen.

Marshall J, Hawrysio A: Inpatient recovery following myocardial infarction and coronary artery bypass graft surgery, *Journal of Cardiovascular Nursing* 2(3):1-12, 1988.

Moore M: *Pocket guide to nutrition and diet therapy,* St Louis, 1988, Mosby.

National Education Programs working group report on the management of patients with hypertension and high blood cholesterol, *Annals of Internal Medicine* 114(3):224-237, 1991.

Redman B: *The process of patient teaching in nursing,* St Louis, 1993, Mosby.

Swearingen P, Keen J, editors: *Manual of critical care,* St Louis, 1991, Mosby.

APPENDIX A

Nursing Diagnoses with Cardiovascular Implications

Standard II from the Standards of Cardiovascular Nursing Practice* addresses nursing diagnoses. Diagnoses are derived from patient health status data, which includes, but is not limited to, history, current medical diagnosis and therapy, psychosocial response to illness, and clinical assessment of cardiovascular status. The following nursing diagnoses are common in patients with cardiovascular disorders.

Nursing Diagnoses	Defining Characteristics	Cardiovascular Related Causes
Circulation		
Decreased cardiac output	Hypotension, tachycardia, restlessness, cyanosis, dyspnea, angina, oliguria, dysrhythmia, fatigability, dizziness, edema	Dysrhythmias, congestive heart failure, cardiogenic shock, cardiac tamponade, myocardial infarction, medications, aortic dissection, pacemaker dysfunction

*From American Nurses' Association on Medical-Surgical Nursing Practice and American Heart Association Council of Cardiovascular Nursing: *Standards of cardiovascular nursing practice,* Kansas City, 1981, American Nurses' Association.

Nursing Diagnoses	Defining Characteristics	Cardiovascular Related Causes
Altered tissue perfusion, peripheral	Claudication; pain at rest, diminished or absent pulse; changes in skin color: pallor, cyanosis, rubor; changes in skin temperature (e.g., coolness); decreased ankle pressure (ankle/arm index <1.0); capillary refill >3 seconds	Peripheral vascular occlusive disease, cardiogenic shock, thromboembolism, vascular trauma, hypertension
Fluid volume deficit	Output > intake, increased serum sodium, dry skin and mucous membranes, tachycardia, hypotension, decreased urinary output, weight loss, hemoconcentration, decreased skin turgor	Cardiac surgery, diuretic therapy
Fluid volume excess	Increased central venous pressure, neck vein distention, S_3, intake > output, edema, taut and shiny skin	Congestive heart failure, myocardial infarction, tachydysrhythmias, cardiopulmonary bypass
Ventilation		
Ineffective airway clearance	Ineffective cough; inability to remove airway secretions; abnormal breath sounds; altered respiratory rate, rhythm, and depth	Anesthesia, bedrest and decreased mobility, medication, incisional pain, infection

Continued.

Nursing Diagnoses	Defining Characteristics	Cardiovascular Related Causes
Ineffective breathing pattern	Change in respiratory rate or pattern from baseline, change in heart rate or rhythm from baseline, orthopnea	Anesthesia, intubation, bedrest and decreased mobility, pleural effusion, pneumothorax/hemothorax, congestive heart failure, anxiety or fear related to pain or prognosis
Impaired gas exchange	Dyspnea, fatigue, increased pulmonary vascular resistance, decreased Pao_2 and O_2 saturation, increased $Paco_2$, cyanosis	Anesthesia, intubation, cardiopulmonary bypass, bedrest and decreased mobility, atelectasis, pulmonary embolism, pulmonary edema
Comfort		
Pain	Patient complains of pain; increase in pulse, blood pressure, respiration; evidence of inflammation; tense body posture, guarded positioning	Angina, myocardial infarction, incisional pain, pericarditis, tissue trauma, immobility
Mobility		
Activity intolerance	Dyspnea, shortness of breath, bradycardia, tachycardia (>20 bpm above resting rate), failure of systolic blood pressure to increase with activity, increase in diastolic blood pressure (>10 mm Hg above resting), weakness, fatigue, dizziness	Congestive heart failure, dysrhythmias, angina or myocardial infarction, hypovolemia, endocarditis

Nursing Diagnoses	Defining Characteristics	Cardiovascular Related Causes
Nutrition		
Altered nutrition, less than body requirements	Food intake < recommended daily allowance (RDA), metabolic needs > intake, weight < ideal	Intubation; medication; ileus; lack of appetite; stress, anxiety, and depression; congestive heart failure; fatigue; dislike of restricted diet
Elimination		
Constipation	Patient cannot move bowels; stools are hard and formed, defecation is strained and painful	Medication, decreased mobility, ileus
Diarrhea	Loose, liquid stools; increased bowel movements	Complications of AAA resection, medication
Sleep and Rest		
Sleep pattern disturbance	Difficulty falling or remaining asleep, napping during the day, mood alterations	Medication, dyspnea, pain, noise, anxiety, depression, unfamiliar environment
Sexuality		
Sexual dysfunction	Patient states difficulty, limitation, or change in sexual function	Medication, peripheral vascular occlusive disease, anxiety or stress, fear of angina or myocardial infarction, altered self-concept

Continued.

Nursing Diagnoses	Defining Characteristics	Cardiovascular Related Causes
Skin Integrity		
Impaired skin integrity	Disruption of skin integrity, erythema, lesions, pruritus	Peripheral vascular occlusive disease, invasive lines, surgical incisions, bedrest and decreased mobility, edema
Education		
Knowledge deficit	Patient requests information, patient discusses inaccurate information, patient inaccurately performs a desired or prescribed health behavior, patient exhibits anxiety or depression	Hospitalization, diagnosis or prognosis, lifestyle changes, discharge needs, medications, diet changes, activity changes
Safety		
High risk for injury	Favorable conditions and risk factors	ICU environment and hospitalization, pacemaker, medication, invasive lines, mental confusion
Infection		
High risk for infection	Favorable conditions or risk factors	Invasive lines and procedures, debilitated state, surgical incisions, immunosuppression, valvular disease

Normal Adult Hemodynamic Values

Parameter	Range*
Pressures (mm Hg)	
Arterial, brachial	
Systolic	100-140
Diastolic	60-90
Mean (MAP) =	70-105
$\dfrac{\text{systolic} + (\text{diastolic} \times 2)}{3}$	
or ⅓ pulse pressure + diastolic pressure	
Left atrial	4-12
Left ventricular	
Systolic	100-140
Diastolic	4-12
Pulmonary artery	
Systolic	15-30
Diastolic	5-15
Mean (PAM)	10-20
Wedge (PAWP)	4-12
Right atrial (CVP)	0-8 (2-12 cm H_2O)
Right ventricular	
Systolic	15-28
Diastolic	0-8

*Ranges may vary depending on source.
CVP, central venous pressure.

Parameter	Range*
Other Values	
Cardiac index (CI) = CO/BSA (CO adjusted for body surface area)	2.8-4.2 L/min/m^2
Cardiac output (CO) = HR × SV (amount of blood ejected into systemic circulation per min)	4-8 L/min
Ejection fraction (EF) = SV/EDV × 100 (percentage of ventricular volume ejected with each contraction)	>60%
Left ventricular stroke work index (LVSWI) = (MAP-PAD)SV × 0.0136/ BSA (index of LV contractility adjusted for body size)	35-85 gm/m^2/beat
Pulmonary vascular resistance (PVR) = PAM − PAWP/CO × 80 (measure of impedance in pulmonary vascular system [RV afterload])	45-120 dyne/sec/ cm^{-5}
Pulmonary vascular resistance index (PVRI) = PAM − PAWP/CI × 80 (measure of RV afterload adjusted for body size)	200-450 dyne/sec/ cm^{-5}
Pulse pressure = systolic pressure − diastolic pressure (reflects stroke volume)	30-40 mm Hg
Rate pressure product (RPP) = HR × systolic pressure (index of myocardial oxygen consumption)	<12,000
Stroke volume (SV) = CO/HR (amount of blood ejected from ventricle with each contraction)	60-100 ml/beat
Stroke volume index (SVI) = SV/BSA (SV adjusted for body surface area)	35-70 ml/m^2/beat

*Ranges may vary depending on source.
EDV, end diastolic volume. HR, heart rate.

Parameter	Range*
Systemic vascular resistance (SVR) = MAP − CVP/CO × 80 (measure of impedance in systemic vascular system [LV afterload])	900-1600 dyne/sec/cm^{-5}
Systemic vascular resistance index (SVRI) = MAP − CVP/CI × 80 (measure of LV afterload adjusted for body size)	1700-2600 dyne/sec/cm^{-5}

*Ranges may vary depending on source.

APPENDIX C
Guide to Cardiac Output Assessment

Normal Values

Parameter	Range*
CI	2.8-4.2 L/min/m^2
CO	4-8 L/min
CVP	0-8 mm Hg
HR	60-100 bpm
LVSWI	35-85 g/m^2/beat
MAP	70-105 mm Hg
PAM	10-20 mm Hg
PAP	15-30 mm Hg
	5-15 mm Hg
PAWP	4-12 mm Hg
PP	30-40 mm Hg
SBP	>100 < 140 mm Hg
SVI	35-70 ml/m^2/beat
Svo$_2$	60%-80%
SVR	900-1600 dyne/sec/cm^{-5}
SVRI	1700-2600 dyne/sec/cm^{-5}

CI, cardiac index. CO, cardiac output. CVP, central venous pressure. HR, heart rate. bpm, beats per minute. LVSWI, left ventricular stroke work index. MAP, mean arterial pressure. PAM, pulmonary artery mean pressure. PAP, pulmonary artery pressure. PAWP, pulmonary artery wedge pressure. PP, pulse pressure. SBP, systolic blood pressure. SVI, stroke volume index. Svo$_2$, mixed venous oxygen saturation. SVR, systemic vascular resistance. SVRI, systemic vascular resistance index.

Evidence of Acute Decreased CO*

Physical signs:	↓Cerebral perfusion—restless, confused, irritable
	↓Peripheral perfusion—mottled, dusky, cyanotic, cool, moist skin; diminished, weak, absent pulses; capillary refill > 3 sec
	↓Renal perfusion—<0.5 ml/kg/hr urine output
Hemodynamic signs:	SBP < 80 mm Hg
	MAP < 60 mm Hg
	HR > 110 or < 50 bpm
	CI < 2.0 L/min/m^2
	CO < 5 L/min
	CVP† < 2 mm Hg or > 8 mm Hg
	PP < 30 mm Hg
	PAP† < $\frac{15}{5}$ mm Hg or > $\frac{30}{15}$ mm Hg
	PAWP < 4 mm Hg or > 18 mm Hg
	SVR < 800 or > 1600 dyne/sec/cm^{-5}
	SVRI < 1700 or > 2600 dyne/sec/cm^{-5}
	LVSWI < 35 g/m^2/beat
	Svo$_2$ < 60% or > 80%

*Trends are more significant than single one-time measurements.
†If CVP (RAP) and LAP (PAD) are elevated, suspect hypervolemia or tamponade. If CVP (RAP) and LAP (PAD) are decreased, suspect hypovolemia. If CVP (RAP) is low and LAP, PAD, or PAWP is elevated, suspect LV dysfunction.

Common Causes and Treatment of Decreased Cardiac Output

Cause	Treatment
Preload, Decreased Hypovolemia (excessive diuresis, hemorrhage) Excessive vasodilation (vasodilator therapy)	Administer fluids, treat cause, administer vasopressor agents
Preload, Increased Volume overload Cardiac failure Valvular insufficiency Mitral/pulmonic stenosis Cardiogenic shock	Diuretic agents, vasodilators

Impedance to diastolic filling:
 	
    Cardiac tamponade
    PEEP
    RV infarction
    Tachydysrhythmias
	Provide volume; treat cause (pericardiocentesis, ventilator changes, antidysrhythmic agents, pacemaker)

Contractility, Decreased Cardiac failure Cardiogenic shock	Inotropic agents
Afterload, Decreased Excessive vasodilation	Treat cause (nitrate, vasodilator therapy), administer vasopressor agents
Afterload, Increased Hypertension Aortic stenosis	Arterial vasodilator agents, IABP

IABP, intra-aortic balloon pump.

APPENDIX D

Conversion Factors/Table of Equivalent Values

Conversion Factors

From	To	Multiply By
cm H_2O	mm Hg	0.735
mm Hg	cm H_2O	1.36
mg	μg	1000
μg	mg	0.100
pound	kilogram	0.4536
kilogram	pound	2.2
centigrade	fahrenheit	1.8 (then add 32)
fahrenheit	centigrade	(subtract 32) then multiply by 0.5555
PSI (pounds/square inch)	mm Hg	51.71
mm Hg	PSI	0.193
inch	cm	2.54

Table of Equivalent Values

1 kilogram (kg) = 1000 grams (g)	1 g = 15 grains (gr)
1 g = 1000 milligrams (mg)	1 gr = 60 mg
1 mg = 0.001 g	1/100 gr = 0.6 mg
1 mg = 1000 micrograms (μg)	1/150 gr = 0.4 mg
	1 teaspoon = 5 milliliters (ml)
1 μg = 0.001 mg	1 tablespoon = 15 ml
1 oz = 30 g	2 tablespoons = 30 ml
	30 ml = 1 ounce (oz)

APPENDIX E
Drug Calculations

Conversion of Grams and Milligrams to Micrograms

Most drug dosages are expressed as milligrams (mg) or micrograms (μg).

To convert milligrams to micrograms, multiply the number of milligrams by 1000

$$mg \times 1000 = \mu g$$

Example: 5 mg

$$5 \times 1000 = 5000 \ \mu g$$

To convert grams to milligrams, multiply the number of grams by 1000

$$g \times 1000 = mg$$

Example: 1.5 g

$$1.5 \times 1000 = 1500 \ mg$$

Drug Concentration—mg/ml or μg/ml

Most drug concentrations are expressed as milligrams per milliliter (mg/ml) or micrograms per milliliter (μg/ml).

To determine the drug concentration, divide the amount of medication by the amount of solution.

$$\frac{\text{Amount of drug (g, mg, or } \mu \text{g})}{\text{Amount of solution (ml)}}$$

Example: 2 mg epinephrine in 250 ml D_5W

    1. Change mg to μg

      $2 \times 1000 = 2000 \ \mu g$

    2. Divide the drug dosage by the amount of solution

$$\frac{2000 \ \mu g}{250 \ ml} = 8 \ \mu g/ml$$

Calculating $\mu g/kg/min$

Many drug concentrations are expressed as micrograms per kilogram per minute ($\mu g/kg/min$), or the amount of drug the patient is receiving per minute based on body weight.

To determine the amount of medication the patient is receiving, three factors must be determined:

1. Drug concentration ($\mu g/ml$)
2. Infusion rate (ml/hr)
3. Patient weight in kg (divide weight in pounds by 2.2)

Multiply the drug concentration by the infusion rate and divide by patient weight $\times$ 60 min/hr.

$$\frac{\mu g/ml \times ml/hr}{kg \times 60 \ min/hr} = \mu g/kg/min$$

Example: 400 mg dopamine in 250 ml D_5W infusing at 60 ml/hr in a patient who weighs 154 pounds

    1. Determine drug concentration

$$\frac{amount \ of \ drug \ (\mu g)}{amount \ of \ solution \ (ml)}$$

      First, convert mg to μg

      $400 \ mg \times 1000 = 400,000 \ \mu g$

      Then, divide the dosage in μg by the amount of solution in milliliters

$$\frac{400000 \ \mu g}{250 \ ml} = 1600 \ \mu g/ml$$

    2. Determine infusion rate (ml/hr): 60 ml/hr

    3. Determine patient weight in kg: (divide pounds by 2.2)

$$\frac{154}{2.2} = 70 \ kg$$

Continued.

Finally,

$$\frac{\mu g/ml \times ml/hr}{kg \times 60 \; min/hr} = \mu g/kg/min$$

$$\frac{1600 \times 60}{70 \times 60} = 23 \; \mu g/kg/min$$

Calculating the Infusion Rate (ml/hr)

To determine the infusion rate for the IV controller pump, three factors must be determined:

1. Dose ordered by the physician (μg/kg/min)
2. Patient weight in kg
3. Drug concentration (μg/ml of IV mixture)

Multiply the dose ordered $\times$ the patient's weight $\times$ 60 min and divide by the drug concentration.

$$\frac{\mu g \; ordered \times kg \times 60 \; min}{\mu g/ml} = ml/hr$$

Example: A patient weighing 165 pounds is to receive dobutamine at 5 μg/kg/min. The drug concentration is 250 mg in 250 ml D_5W.

1. Dose ordered is 5 μg/kg/min

2. Determine patient weight in kg (divide pounds by 2.2)

$$\frac{165}{2.2} = 75 \; kg$$

3. Determine drug concentration in μg/ml

   First, convert mg to μg:

   250 mg $\times$ 1000 = 250,000 μg

Then divide the drug dosage by the amount of solution

$$\frac{250,000 \; \mu g}{250 \; ml} = 1000 \; \mu g/ml$$

Finally,

$$\frac{\mu g \times kg \times 60 \; min}{\mu g/ml} = ml/hr$$

$$\frac{5 \times 75 \times 60}{1000} = 22\text{-}23 \; ml/hr$$

Therapeutic Serum Levels of Select Cardiovascular Drugs

Drugs	Therapeutic Level*
Amiodarone	0.5-2.5 μg/ml
Bretylium tosylate	0.5-1.5 μg/ml
Digoxin	0.5-2.0 ng/ml
Digitoxin	5.0-30 ng/ml
Disopyramide	2.0-8.0 μg/ml
Flecainide	0.2-1.0 μg/ml
Lidocaine	1.5-6.0 μg/ml
Mexiletine	0.5-2.0 μg/ml
Nitroprusside†	
thiocyanate	100 μg/ml
cyanide	3 μmol/ml
N-acetyl-procainamide (NAPA)	10-20 μg/ml
Procainamide	4.0-8.0 μg/ml
Propafenone	0.06-1.0 μg/ml
Propranolol	0.05-0.1 μg/ml
Quinidine	2.0-6.0 μg/ml
Tocainide	4.0-10 μg/ml
Verapamil	0.08-0.3 μg/ml

*Levels may vary depending upon source.
†Toxic levels.

APPENDIX G

Drugs Commonly Used in a Cardiovascular Emergency

Drug dosages are based on ACLS standards.

Drug	Indications	Dosage	Clinical Alert
First-Line Code Drugs*			
Atropine sulfate	Bradycardia associated with hypo-tension, dys-rhythmia, or myocardial ischemia	*IV:* 0.5-1.0 mg; repeat q 3-5 min; up to 0.04 mg/kg	Give over 1 minute; DO NOT EXCEED 0.04 mg/kg; 2-2.5 × the recommended IV dose can be given
	Asystole	*IV:* 1.0 mg; repeat q 3-5 min up to 0.04 mg/kg	endotracheally—give in 10 ml NS; follow with forceful inhala-tions. VF and VT can occur.
Dopamine (Intropin)	Hypotension	*Infusion:* 2.5-20 μg/kg/min	800 mg diluted in 500 ml D_5W yields 1600 μg/ml. Check BP q 2-5 min dur-ing titration. Monitor ECG for ventricular

*Refer to ACLS algorithms (Appendix H).

Drug	Indications	Dosage	Clinical Alert
			dysrhythmias and widening QRS complex. Extravasation can result in tissue necrosis.* Taper dosage slowly.
Epinephrine (Adrenalin)	VF, pulseless VT, asystole, EMD Symptomatic bradycardia	*IV*: 1.0 mg; repeat q 3-5 min *Infusion:* 1 μg/min; titrate to desired response	During cardiac arrest: 30 mg in 250 ml D_5W; run at 100 ml/hr and titrate to desired effect. As a vasopressor agent: 1 mg in 500 ml D_5W; 1 μg/min = 30 ml/hr. 2-2.5 × the recommended IV dose may be given endotracheally—give in 10 ml NS; follow with forceful inhalations. Monitor for ventricular ectopy. Check BP q 2 to 5 min during titration. Do not give with isoproterenol.

*To prevent tissue necrosis, administer 5-10 mg phentolamine (Regitine) diluted in 10-15 ml of NS into tissue via a large gauge needle.

Drug	Indications	Dosage	Clinical Alert
Lidocaine (Xylocaine)	VT, VF, PVCs	*IV:* 1-1.5 mg/kg; Repeat 0.5-1.5 mg/kg q 5-10 min up to 3 mg/kg *Infusion:* 2-4 mg/min. Do not exceed 4 mg/min	Bolus dose: 1.0-1.5 mg/kg over 1 min. Reduce dosage in elderly and those with liver impairment. 2 g in 500 ml D_5W yields 4 mg/ml 1 mg/min = 15 ml/hr 2 mg/min = 30 ml/hr 3 mg/min = 45 ml/hr 4 mg/min = 60 ml/hr Monitor ECG and BP. DO NOT EXCEED an infusion rate of 4 mg/min.
Other Drugs Adenosine (Adenocard)	PSVT	IV: 6 mg over 1 to 2 sec. If PSVT is not eliminated within 1-2 min, give 12 mg rapidly IV. Repeat 12 mg dose a second time if needed.	After bolus, flush with 20 ml saline. Monitor ECG for prolonged PR interval. Dysrhythmias may occur when PSVT converts to sinus rhythm. Heart blocks are generally self-limiting.

Drug	Indications	Dosage	Clinical Alert
			Check patient for nonmyo-cardial chest discomfort, hypotension, or dyspnea.
Alteplase (Activase)	Coronary artery thrombosis	*IV:* * 6-10 mg over 2 min, followed by 50-54 mg over the first hr and 20 mg/hr for 2 hours. Patients <65 kg should receive a total dose of 1.25 mg/kg; three fifths of the total dose should be divided between a bolus and first hour dose; then give one fifth dose over the second hour and the last one fifth dose over the third hour.	Obtain CK, CK-MB, and clotting studies. Do not use a filter. Do not mix with any other drug. At the completion of the infusion, clear the IV tubing with at least 30 ml of NS or D_5W and run at 1 ml/min to ensure total dose of alteplase is given. Monitor ECG for ST changes, dysrhythmias. Check patient for bleeding and chest pain.
Amrinone (Inocor)	Cardiac failure refractory to conventional therapy	*IV:* 0.75 mg/kg over 2-3 min. *Infusion:* 5-15 μg/kg/min	100 mg in 100 ml NS yields 1 mg/ml. Do not mix with dextrose solutions.

---

*Recommended by manufacturer.   *Continued.*

Drug	Indications	Dosage	Clinical Alert
			Use lowest necessary dose to achieve desired response. Monitor hemodynamic status: CO, CI, PAP, BP. Monitor ECG for dysrhythmias.
Anistreplase (Eminase)	Coronary artery thrombosis	*IV:* 30 units over 2-5 min	Must be used within 30 min of reconstitution. Stop the flow of IV fluids during anistreplase injection. Flush IV line after injection. Do not mix with any other drug. Check patient for allergic reaction. Monitor ECG for ST changes, dysrhythmias. Monitor BP.
Bretylium tosylate (Bretylol)	Ventricular dysrhythmia unresponsive to lidocaine and procainamide	*IV:* 5 mg/kg; increase to 10 mg/kg and repeat q 5 min. *Infusion:* 1-2 mg/min	Wait 1-2 min before defibrillation. Maximum dose is 30-35 mg/kg. Can produce high

Drug	Indications	Dosage	Clinical Alert
			blood pressure and tachycardia initially. Hypotension is common; keep patient supine. Monitor BP and ECG. 2 g in 500 ml D_5W yields 4 mg/ml. 1 mg/min = 15 ml/hr 2 mg/min = 30 ml/hr
Calcium chloride	Acute hyperkalemia, hypocalcemia; calcium channel blocker toxicity	*IV:* 2-4 mg/kg of 10% solution; Repeat in 10 min if needed	Do not give with sodium bicarbonate. Watch for bradycardia. Ventricular irritability can occur in patients receiving digitalis. Extravasation can result in tissue necrosis.
Digoxin (Lanoxin)	Cardiac failure, atrial flutter, atrial fibrillation	*Digitalization:* single IV dose of 0.5-0.75 mg *Maintenance:* 0.125-0.5 mg/day	Administer IV dose over 5 min; can be given undiluted. Check serum potassium level;

Continued.

Drug	Indications	Dosage	Clinical Alert
			myocardium is sensitive to digitalis intoxication if hypokalemia exists. Monitor ECG for ST segment sagging, prolongation of PR interval, or dysrhythmias. Many drugs potentiate digoxin levels (i.e., esmolol, quinidine, verapamil, propranolol).
Dobutamine (Dobutrex)	Cardiac failure, cardiogenic shock	*Infusion:* 2.0-20 µg/kg/min; titrate to desired response	500 mg in 250 ml D_5W yields 2000 µg/ml. Use lowest dose possible. Watch for dysrhythmias or changes in BP. Monitor CO, PAWP.
Esmolol (Brevibloc)	Supraventricular tachycardia	500 µg/kg/min for 1 min, then 50 µg/kg/min for 4 min. Repeat loading dose and increase infusion to	5 g in 500 ml D_5W yields 10 mg/ml. Esmolol must be diluted with 20 ml of the total amount of

Drug	Indications	Dosage	Clinical Alert
		100 µg/kg/min if desired response is not achieved within 5 min. Continue same loading dose but increase the maintenance dose by 50 µg/kg/min until desired response is achieved or hypotension occurs. DO NOT EXCEED 200 µg/kg/min.	500 D_5W solution before adding it to the remaining 480 ml. Monitor BP every 2 min during titration. Monitor ECG for dysrhythmia control.
Furosemide (Lasix)	Cardiac failure, pulmonary edema	*IV:* 0.5-1.0 mg/kg initially	Administer 20 mg over 1 min. Transient deafness can result with high doses. Monitor for hypovolemia, dysrhythmias, hypokalemia, circulatory collapse. Measure urine output.

Continued.

Drug	Indications	Dosage	Clinical Alert
Heparin	Prevention of clot formation, thrombosis, emboli	Determined with clotting studies. Usual dosage: 20,000-40,000 units/24 hours	Can be given undiluted. A bolus of 5000-10,000 U is usually required initially. Monitor activated partial thromboplastin time. Watch for bleeding. Avoid invasive procedures.
Isoproterenol (Isuprel)	Temporary control of hemodynamic significant bradycardia in the denervated heart (transplant); and in refractory torsades de pointes until pacemaker therapy is initiated.	*Infusion:* 2-10 μg/min; titrate to pulse of 60	1 mg in 500 ml D_5W yields 2 μg/ml. 1 μg/min = 30 ml/hr 2 μg/min = 60 ml/hr 3 μg/min = 90 ml/hr 4 μg/min = 120 ml/hr 5 μg/min = 150 ml/hr Contraindicated in cardiac arrest. Monitor for dysrhythmias, ischemia, tachycardia. Do not use in conjunction with epinephrine.

Drug	Indications	Dosage	Clinical Alert
Magnesium	Hypomagnesemia	*IV loading dose*: 1-2 g/50-100 ml D_5W; give over 5-60 min; follow with 0.5-1.0 g/hr for 24 hr	Monitor ECG for response to treatment
	VF/VT	1-2 g/100 ml D_5W over 1-2 min.	
	Torsades de pointes	1-2 g/100 ml D_5W over 1-2 min; follow with 1-2 g/100 ml D_5W over 1 hr.	
Morphine sulfate	Angina, pulmonary edema	*IV:* 1-3 mg q 5 min.	Dilute with at least 5 ml NS or sterile water. Administer over 4-5 min. Monitor respirations (do not give if <10/min), HR, BP. Keep naloxone (Narcan) on hand.
Nitroglycerin	Cardiac failure, angina	*Infusion:* 5 μg/min; increase by 5-10 μg/min q 5-10 min. Titrate to desired response. No maximum dose established	50 mg in 500 ml D_5W yields 100 μg/ml. 5 μg/min = 3 ml/hr 10 μg/min = 6 ml/hr Do not mix with other

Continued.

Drug	Indications	Dosage	Clinical Alert
			drugs. Use special IV tubing and glass container. Monitor BP q 2-5 min during titration. Stop infusion if hypotension occurs.
Norepinephrine (Levophed)	Hypotension refractory to other drugs	*Infusion:* 0.5-1.0 µg/min initially; titrate to desired effect	4 mg in 250 ml D_5W yields 16 µg/ml. 1 µg/min = 4 ml/hr 2 µg/min = 8 ml/hr 3 µg/min = 12 ml/hr Use on a temporary basis. Monitor BP q 2-5 min. Monitor for dysrhythmias. Extravasation results in tissue necrosis.
Phytonadione (Aquamephyton-vitamin K)	Antidote for warfarin	*IV:* 2.5-25 mg over 1 min	IV route for emergency use only. Watch for hypotension, diaphoresis, dyspnea,

Drug	Indications	Dosage	Clinical Alert
			flushing, peculiar taste in mouth.
Potassium chloride	Hypokalemia	20-60 mEq/24 hr, up to 400 mEq/24 hr	NEVER GIVE IV PUSH. GIVE DILUTED. DO NOT EXCEED 10 mEq/hr VIA PERIPHERAL VEIN. Monitor ECG. Do not give to anuric patients. Extravasation can result in tissue necrosis.
Procainamide (Pronestyl)	Ventricular dysrhythmia unresponsive to lidocaine	*IV:* 20 mg/min up to 17 mg/kg *Infusion:* 1-4 mg/min as a maintenance dose	Give 20 mg over 1 min. Repeat IV dose until dysrhythmia is suppressed, hypotension occurs, QRS widens by 50% of the original width, or 17 mg/kg has been given.

Continued.

Drug	Indications	Dosage	Clinical Alert
			2 g in 500 ml D_5W yields 4 mg/ml. 1 mg/min = 15 ml/hr 2 mg/min = 30 ml/hr 3 mg/min = 45 ml/hr 4 mg/min = 60 ml/hr Monitor ECG, and BP q2-5 min during titration.
Protamine sulfate	Neutralizes anticoagulant effects of heparin	1 mg/100 USP units of heparin; repeat in 10-15 min. DO NOT EXCEED 50 mg in any 10 min period	Administer 20 mg over 1-3 min. Bradycardia, dyspnea, hypotension or hypertension may result from too rapid injection.
Sodium bicarbonate	Metabolic acidosis	1 mEq/kg IV; Repeat ½ the initial dose after 10 min of resuscitation or if pH indicates	Give over 1-3 min. Monitor for hypernatremia and hyperosmolality. Extravasation can result in tissue necrosis. Clear IV line before and after administration.

Drug	Indications	Dosage	Clinical Alert
Sodium nitro-prusside (Nipride)	Cardiac failure, hypertension	*Infusion:* 0.1-5.0 μg/kg/min; titrate to desired response. DO NOT EXCEED 10 μg/kg/min	50 mg in 250 ml D_5W yields 200 μg/ml. Wrap solution in protective aluminum foil. Monitor BP q 1-5 min during titration, then q 15 min. Patients are at risk for thiocyanate toxicity if dosage is >8 μg/kg/min or infusion lasts longer than 2-3 days.
Streptokinase (Streptase)	Coronary artery thrombosis	*IV:* 1,500,000 IU over 1 hour if within 6 hours of onset of symptoms, 750,000 IU over 10 min if within 3 hours of onset of symptoms; follow with 250,000 IU over ½ -1 hour	Dilute 1,500,000 IU in 100 ml or 750,000 IU in 50 ml of NS or D_5W. Do not mix with other drugs. Obtain CK and clotting studies. Diphenhydramine (Benadryl) may be given to reduce risk of allergic reaction. Monitor ECG for ST

Continued.

Drug	Indications	Dosage	Clinical Alert
			changes and dysrhythmias. Monitor for chest pain and bleeding.
Verapamil (Isoptin, Calan)	PSVT	*IV:* 2.5-5 mg; repeat with 5-10 mg q 15-30 min; maximum dosage is 20 mg	Administer over 2 min. Monitor ECG, BP. Monitor for heart failure. Do not administer disopyramide (Norpace) 48 hours before or 24 hours after verapamil. Myocardial depression can occur if verapamil is used in conjunction with beta blocking agents.

APPENDIX H
ACLS Algorithms*

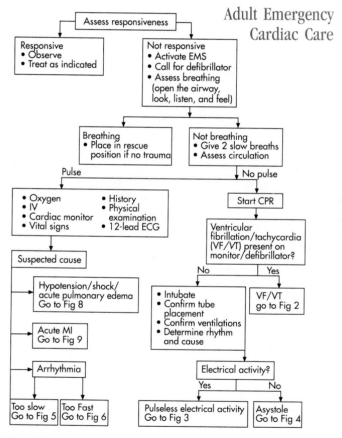

Adult Emergency Cardiac Care

Figure 1
Universal algorithm for adult emergency cardiac care (ECC).

*From Emergency Cardiac Care Committee and Subcommittees, American Heart Association: *JAMA* 268(16):2216-2230, 1992. Copyright 1992, American Medical Association.

317

Ventricular Fibrillation/Pulseless Ventricular Tachycardia

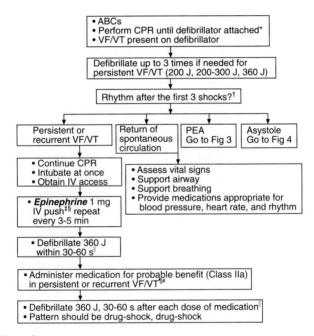

Figure 2
Algorithm for ventricular fibrillation and pulseless ventricular tachycardia (VF/VT).

Class I: definitely helpful
Class IIa: acceptable, probably helpful
Class IIb: acceptable, possibly helpful
Class III: not indicated, may be harmful
*Precordial thump is a Class IIb action in witnessed arrest, no pulse, and no defibrillator immediately available.
†Hypothermic cardiac arrest is treated differently after this point. See section on hypothermia.
‡The recommended dose of **epinephrine** is 1 mg IV push every 3-5 min. If this approach fails, several Class IIb dosing regimens can be considered:
• Intermediate: **epinephrine** 2-5 mg IV push, every 3-5 min
• Escalating: **epinephrine** 1 mg-3 mg-5 mg IV push (3 min apart)
• High: **epinephrine** 0.1 mg/kg IV push, every 3-5 min
§**Sodium bicarbonate** (1 mEq/kg) is Class I if patient has known pre-existing hyperkalemia
‖Multiple sequenced shocks (200 J, 200-300 J, 360 J) are acceptable here (Class I), especially when medications are delayed

¶• **Lidocaine** 1.5 mg/kg IV push. Repeat in 3-5 min to total loading dose of 3 mg/kg; then use
• **Bretylium** 5 mg/kg IV push. Repeat in 5 min at 10 mg/kg
• **Magnesium sulfate** 1-2 g IV in torsades de pointes or suspected hypomagnesemic state or severe refractory VF
• **Procainamide** 30 mg/min in refractory VF (maximum total 17 mg/kg)
#• **Sodium bicarbonate** (1 mEq/kg IV):
Class IIa
• if known preexisting bicarbonate-responsive acidosis
• if overdose with tricyclic antidepressants
• to alkalinize the urine in drug overdoses
Class IIb
• if intubated and continued long arrest interval
• upon return of spontaneous circulation after long arrest interval
Class III
• hypoxic lactic acidosis

Pulseless Electrical Activity

PEA includes

- Electromechanical dissociation (EMD)
- Pseudo-EMD
- Idioventricular rhythms
- Ventricular escape rhythms
- Bradyasystolic rhythms
- Postdefibrillation idioventricular rhythms

- Continue CPR
- Intubate at once
- Obtain IV access
- Assess blood flow using Doppler ultrasound

Consider possible causes
(Parentheses=possible therapies and treatments)
- Hypovolemia (volume infusion)
- Hypoxia (ventilation)
- Cardiac tamponade (pericardiocentesis)
- Tension pneumothorax (needle decompression)
- Hypothermia (see hypothermia algorithm, Section IV)
- Massive pulmonary embolism (surgery, **thrombolytics**)
- Drug overdoses such as tricyclics, digitalis, β-blockers, calcium channel blockers
- Hyperkalemia*
- Acidosis†
- Massive acute myocardial infarction (go to Fig 9)

- **Epinephrine** 1 mg IV push, *†repeat every 3-5 min

- If absolute bradycardia (<60 beats/min) or relative bradycardia, give **atropine** 1 mg IV
- Repeat every 3-5 min up to a total of 0.04 mg/kg§

Figure 3
Algorithm for pulseless electrical activity (PEA) (electromechanical dissociation [EMD]).

Class I: definitely helpful
Class IIa: acceptable, probably helpful
Class IIb: acceptable, possibly helpful
Class III: not indicated, may be harmful
*__Sodium bicarbonate__ 1 mEq/kg is Class I if patient has known preexisting hyperkalemia
†__Sodium bicarbonate__ 1 mEq/kg:
Class IIa
- if known preexisting bicarbonate-responsive acidosis
- if overdose with tricyclic antidepressants
- to alkalinize the urine in drug overdoses
   Class IIb
- if intubated and long arrest interval
- upon return of spontaneous circulation after long arrest interval
   Class III
- hypoxic lactic acidosis
†The recommended dose of __epinephrine__ is 1 mg IV push every 3-5 min.
If this approach fails, several Class IIb dosing regimens can be considered.
- Intermediate: __epinephrine__ 2-5 mg IV push, every 3-5 min
- Escalating: __epinephrine__ 1 mg-3 mg-5 mg IVpush (3 min apart)
- High: __epinephrine__ 0.1 mg/kg IV push, every 3-5 min
§Shorter __atropine__ dosing intervals possibly helpful in cardiac arrest (Class IIb).

Asystole

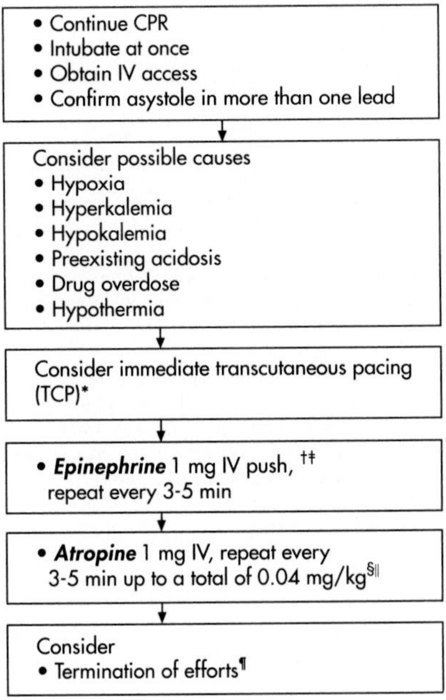

Figure 4
Asystole treatment algorithm.

Class I: definitely helpful
Class IIa: acceptable, probably helpful
Class IIb: acceptable, possibly helpful
Class III: not indicated, may be harmful

*TCP is a Class IIb intervention. Lack of success may be due to delays in pacing. To be effective TCP must be performed early, simultaneously with drugs. Evidence does not support routine use of TCP for asystole.

†The recommended dose of *epinephrine* is 1 mg IV push every 3-5 min. If this approach fails, several Class IIb dosing regimens can be considered:
- Intermediate: *epinephrine* 2-5 mg IV push, every 3-5 min
- Escalating: *epinephrine* 1 mg-3 mg-5 mg IV push (3 min apart)
- High: *epinephrine* 0.1 mg/kg IV push, every 3-5 min

‡*Sodium bicarbonate* 1 mEq/kg is Class I if patient has known preexisting hyperkalemia.

§Shorter *atropine* dosing intervals are Class IIb in asystolic arrest.

‖*Sodium bicarbonate* 1 mEq/kg:
Class IIa
- if known preexisting bicarbonate-responsive acidosis
- if overdose with tricyclic antidepressants
- to alkalinize the urine in drug overdoses

Class IIb
- if intubated and continued long arrest interval
- upon return of spontaneous circulation after long arrest interval

Class III
- hypoxic lactic acidosis

¶If patient remains in asystole or other agonal rhythms after successful intubation and initial medications and no reversible causes are identified, consider termination of resuscitative efforts by a physician. Consider interval since arrest.

Bradycardia

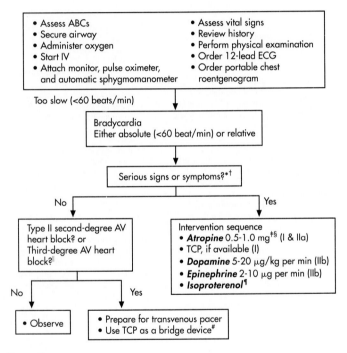

Figure 5
Bradycardia algorithm (with the patient not in cardiac arrest).

*Serious signs or symptoms must be related to the slow rate.
Clinical manifestations include:
symptoms (chest pain, shortness of breath, decreased level of conciousness) and
signs (low BP, shock, pulmonary congestion, CHF, acute MI).
†Do not delay TCP while awaiting IV access or for **atropine** to take effect if patient is symptomatic.
‡Denervated transplanted hearts will not respond to **atropine**. Go at once to pacing, **catecholamine** infusion, or both.
§**Atropine** should be given in repeat doses in 3-5 min up to total of 0.04 mg/kg. Consider shorter dosing intervals in severe clinical conditions. It has been suggested that atropine should be used with caution in atrioventricular (AV) block at the His-Purkinje level (type II AV block and new third-degree block with wide QRS complexes) (Class IIb).
‖Never treat third-degree heart block plus ventricular escape beats with **lidocaine**.
¶**Isoproterenol** should be used, if at all, with extreme caution. At low doses it is Class IIb (possibly helpful); at higher doses it is Class III (harmful).
#Verify patient tolerance and mechanical capture. Use analgesia and sedation as needed.

Tachycardia

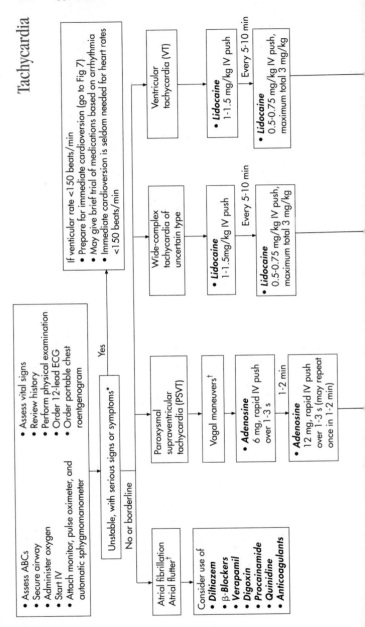

- Assess ABCs
- Secure airway
- Administer oxygen
- Start IV
- Attach monitor, pulse oximeter, and automatic sphygmomanometer
- Assess vital signs
- Review history
- Perform physical examination
- Order 12-lead ECG
- Order portable chest roentgenogram

Unstable, with serious signs or symptoms*

Yes

No or borderline

If ventricular rate <150 beats/min
- Prepare for immediate cardioversion (go to Fig 7)
- May give brief trial of medications based on arrhythmia
- Immediate cardioversion is seldom needed for heart rates <150 beats/min

Ventricular tachycardia (VT)

- *Lidocaine* 1-1.5 mg/kg IV push

Every 5-10 min

- *Lidocaine* 0.5-0.75 mg/kg IV push, maximum total 3 mg/kg

Wide-complex tachycardia of uncertain type

- *Lidocaine* 1-1.5mg/kg IV push

Every 5-10 min

- *Lidocaine* 0.5-0.75 mg/kg IV push, maximum total 3 mg/kg

Paroxysmal supraventricular tachycardia (PSVT)

Vagal maneuvers†

- *Adenosine* 6 mg, rapid IV push over 1-3 s

1-2 min

- *Adenosine* 12 mg, rapid IV push over 1-3 s (may repeat once in 1-2 min)

Atrial fibrillation
Atrial flutter†

Consider use of
- *Diltiazem*
- *β-Blockers*
- *Verapamil*
- *Digoxin*
- *Procainamide*
- *Quinidine*
- *Anticoagulants*

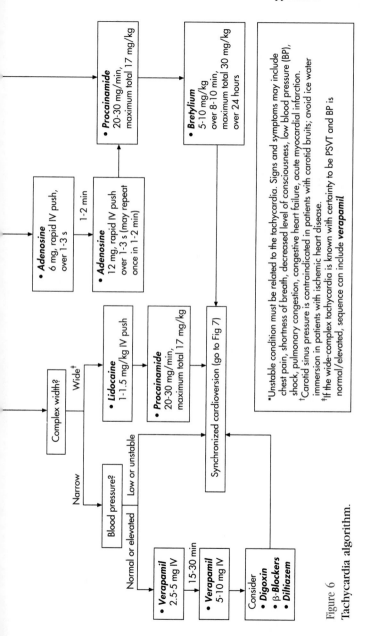

Figure 6
Tachycardia algorithm.

Electrical Cardioversion

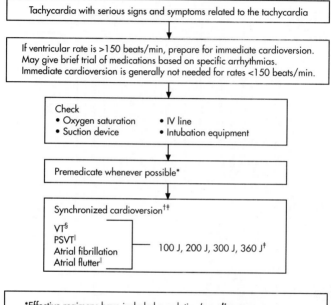

Tachycardia with serious signs and symptoms related to the tachycardia

↓

If ventricular rate is >150 beats/min, prepare for immediate cardioversion. May give brief trial of medications based on specific arrhythmias. Immediate cardioversion is generally not needed for rates <150 beats/min.

↓

Check
- Oxygen saturation
- Suction device
- IV line
- Intubation equipment

↓

Premedicate whenever possible*

↓

Synchronized cardioversion†‡

VT§
PSVT‖
Atrial fibrillation
Atrial flutter‖ ⎯⎯⎯ 100 J, 200 J, 300 J, 360 J†

*Effective regimens have included a sedative (eg, *diazepam, midazolam, barbiturates, etomidate, ketamine, methohexital*) with or without an analgesic agent (e.g., *fentanyl, morphine, meperidine*). Many experts recommend anesthesia if service is readily available.
†Note possible need to resynchronize after each cardioversion.
‡If delays in synchronization occur and clinical conditions are critical, go to immediate unsynchronized shocks.
§Treat polymorphic VT (irregular form and rate) like VF: 200 J, 200-300 J, 360 J.
‖PSVT and atrial flutter often respond to lower energy levels (start with 50 J).

Figure 7
Electrical cardioversion algorithm (with the patient not in cardiac arrest).

Hypotension, Shock, Pulmonary Edema

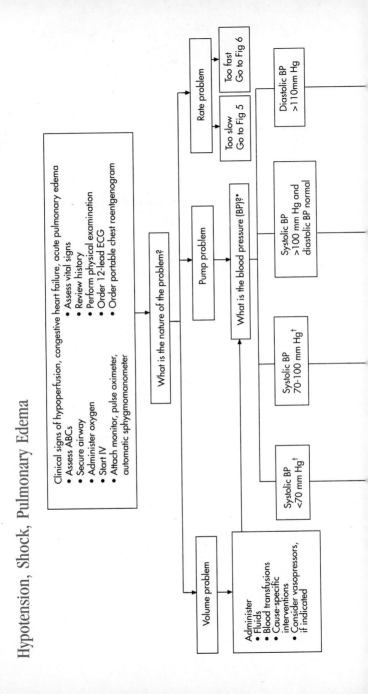

Clinical signs of hypoperfusion, congestive heart failure, acute pulmonary edema

- Assess ABCs
- Secure airway
- Administer oxygen
- Start IV
- Attach monitor, pulse oximeter, automatic sphygmomanometer
- Assess vital signs
- Review history
- Perform physical examination
- Order 12-lead ECG
- Order portable chest roentgenogram

What is the nature of the problem?

Rate problem
- Too slow Go to Fig 5
- Too fast Go to Fig 6

Pump problem

What is the blood pressure (BP)?*

- Systolic BP >100 mm Hg and diastolic BP normal
- Diastolic BP >110 mm Hg
- Systolic BP 70–100 mm Hg†
- Systolic BP <70 mm Hg†

Volume problem

Administer
- Fluids
- Blood transfusions
- Cause-specific interventions
- Consider vasopressors, if indicated

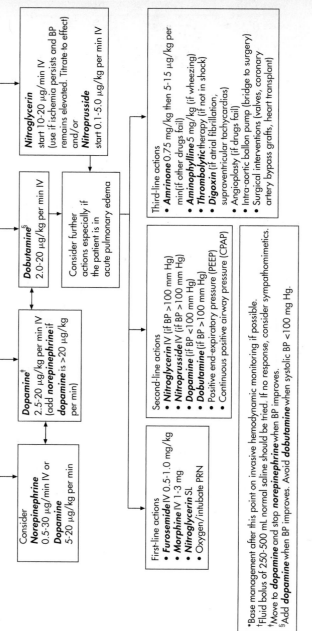

Nitroglycerin
start 10-20 µg/min IV
(use if ischemia persists and BP
remains elevated. Titrate to effect)
and/or
Nitroprusside
start 0.1-5.0 µg/kg per min IV

Dobutamine§
2.0-20 µg/kg per min IV

Dopamine‡
2.5-20 µg/kg per min IV
(add **norepinephrine** if
dopamine is >20 µg/kg
per min)

Consider
Norepinephrine
0.5-30 µg/min IV or
Dopamine
5-20 µg/kg per min

Consider further
actions especially if
the patient is in
acute pulmonary edema

Third-line actions
• **Amrinone** 0.75 mg/kg then 5-15 µg/kg per
  min (if other drugs fail)
• **Aminophylline** 5 mg/kg (if wheezing)
• **Thrombolytic** therapy (if not in shock)
• **Digoxin** (if atrial fibrillation,
  supraventricular tachycardias)
• Angioplasty (if drugs fail)
• Intra-aortic balloon pump (bridge to surgery)
• Surgical interventions (valves, coronary
  artery bypass grafts, heart transplant)

Second-line actions
• **Nitroglycerin** IV (if BP >100 mm Hg)
• **Nitroprusside** IV (if BP >100 mm Hg)
• **Dopamine** (if BP <100 mm Hg)
• **Dobutamine** (if BP >100 mm Hg)
• Positive end-expiratory pressure (PEEP)
• Continuous positive airway pressure (CPAP)

First-line actions
• **Furosemide** IV 0.5-1.0 mg/kg
• **Morphine** IV 1-3 mg
• **Nitroglycerin** SL
• Oxygen/intubate PRN

*Base management after this point on invasive hemodynamic monitoring if possible.
†Fluid bolus of 250-500 mL normal saline should be tried. If no response, consider sympathomimetics.
‡Move to **dopamine** and stop **norepinephrine** when BP improves.
§Add **dopamine** when BP improves. Avoid **dobutamine** when systolic BP <100 mm Hg.

Figure 8
Algorithm for hypotension, shock, and acute pulmonary
edema.

Acute Myocardial Infarction

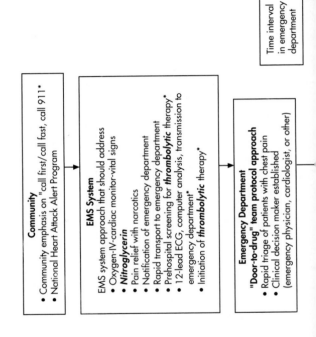

Community
- Community emphasis on "call first/call fast, call 911"*
- National Heart Attack Alert Program

EMS System
EMS system approach that should address
- Oxygen-IV-cardiac monitor-vital signs
- **Nitroglycerin**
- Pain relief with narcotics
- Notification of emergency department
- Rapid transport to emergency department
- Prehospital screening for *thrombolytic* therapy*
- 12-lead ECG, computer analysis, transmission to emergency department*
- Initiation of *thrombolytic* therapy*

Emergency Department
"Door-to-drug" team protocol approach
- Rapid triage of patients with chest pain
- Clinical decision maker established (emergency physician, cardiologist, or other)

Time interval in emergency department

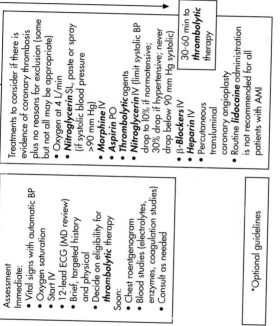

Assessment

Immediate:
- Vital signs with automatic BP
- Oxygen saturation
- Start IV
- 12-lead ECG (MD review)
- Brief, targeted history and physical
- Decide on eligibility for **thrombolytic** therapy

Soon:
- Chest roentgenogram
- Blood studies (electrolytes, enzymes, coagulation studies)
- Consult as needed

Treatments to consider if there is evidence of coronary thrombosis plus no reasons for exclusion (some but not all may be appropriate)
- Oxygen at 4 L/min
- **Nitroglycerin** SL, paste or spray (if systolic blood pressure >90 mm Hg)
- **Morphine** IV
- **Aspirin** PO
- **Thrombolytic** agents
- **Nitroglycerin** IV (limit systolic BP drop to 10% if normotensive; 30% drop if hypertensive; never drop below 90 mm Hg systolic)

- β-**Blockers** IV
- **Heparin** IV
- Percutaneous transluminal coronary angioplasty
- Routine **lidocaine** administration is not recommended for all patients with AMI

30-60 min to **thrombolytic** therapy

*Optional guidelines

Figure 9

Acute myocardial infarction (AMI) algorithm. Recommendations for early treatment of patients with chest pain and possible AMI.

Index

335

Non–Q wave infarction, 7
Nontransmural infarction, 7
Norepinephrine, 160, 312
  precautions with, 163
Normodyne; *see* Labetalol
Norpace; *see* Disopyramide
    phosphate
North American Society of Pacing
    and Electrophysiology, 150
Nuclide venography to diagnose
    thrombophlebitis, 59
Nursing diagnoses with
    cardiovascular
    implications, 286-290
Nylidrin, 228

O

Objective data during
    cardiovascular assessment,
    61
Occlusive disease, peripheral
    vascular; *see* Peripheral
    vascular occlusive disease
Omega-3 fatty acids to retard
    atherosclerosis, 12
Opening snap, 71
Oral contraceptives, lipid levels
    and, 216
Oretic; *see* Hydrochlorothiazide
Orientation, assessment of, 83
Orthopnea, 62
Orthostatic blood pressure, 76
Osler's nodes, 79
Overload, assessment of, 84
Oxygen saturation, mixed venous;
    see Mixed venous oxygen
    saturation
Oxygen therapy, 85
Oxyhemoglobin dissociation
    curve, 93, 95, 97

P

P wave, 101
PAC; *see* Premature atrial
    complex
Pacemaker(s), 148, 150
  malfunction of, 152
  patient education guidelines for,
    277
  permanent, 148

Pacemaker(s)—cont'd
  temporary, 148
  using NBG code, examples of,
    151
Pacemaker code, NBG, 150, 151
PAD; *see* Pulmonary artery
    diastolic pressure
Pain, chest, 62
  differentiating, 63-65
Pallor, 80
Palpitations, 62
PAP; *see* Pulmonary artery
    pressure
Papillary muscle rupture following
    myocardial infarction, 16
Parasympatholytic agent, 168-169
Paroxysmal nocturnal dyspnea, 62
Paroxysmal supraventricular
    tachycardia, 111
Partial thromboplastin time, 91
PAS; *see* Pulmonary artery
    systolic pressure
Patent ductus arteriosus, 41
  auscultatory findings with, 44
Patient, cardiovascular, core
    curriculum for, 259-276
Patient education, 251-258
  about antianginal agents,
    264-266
  about antidysrhythmic agents,
    267-268
  about antihypertensive agents,
    271-272
  about antilipemic agents,
    273-274
  about beta adrenergic blocking
    agents, 265, 266
  about calcium channel blocking
    agents, 265, 266
  about digoxin, 268-269
  about diuretics, 269-270
  documentation of, 257
  about hematologic agents,
    274-275
  about implantable cardioverter
    defibrillators, 278-279
  about nitrates, 264-265, 266
  about pacemakers, 277
  about peripheral vascular
    agents, 275-276